HARD QUESTIONS

SIMPLE ANSWERS

HARD QUESTIONS
SIMPLE ANSWERS

A Workbook for Taking the Crisis out of Caregiving

ELANA PETERS, MA, CMC

SLP

SEVEN LOCKS PRESS

Santa Ana, California
Minneapolis, Minnesota
Washington, D.C.
Helena, Montana

Seven Locks Press,
P.O. Box 25689
Santa Ana, CA 92799
800-354-5348

Printed in the United States of America

ISBN 1-931643-07-5

Library of Congress Cataloging-in-Publication Data is available from the publisher.

Book design by Richard Cheverton/Waypoint

Contents

Introduction

Welcome to one of the most emotional and educational experiences of your lifetime: caregiving for an older adult. Designed to take the crisis out of caregiving, *Hard Questions, Simple Answers* is your guide through the varied and progressive tasks involved in this often unavoidable phase of life.

You will learn a great deal from this stressful and heartbreaking experience, including many ways in which you do not want to grow old.

Hard Questions, Simple Answers systematically outlines the issues and the information you will need to take care of an older adult. Its practical, detailed, and easy-to-use approach enables you to record personal information and pertinent data in a step-by-step manner. Once you have all the information recorded, this workbook will become an invaluable tool when a health-care crisis or medical emergency arises. Keep it easily accessible. This workbook will not only save time for all of those involved in the health-care process-medical personnel, professional-care providers, family members, the older adult-it will simplify and de-stress the process of getting the right information to the right people when it is needed.

Dear Caregiver, do not attempt to complete the information pages in this workbook in a single sitting. This is a process, not a fill-in-the-blanks test. You and your caregiving recipient will probably need to work on it together. Gathering and organizing this data could be the best thing you do for yourself, your family, and the older adult during this time of emotional instability.

Hard Questions, Simple Answers is a beneficial gift to those concerned with health and life-care choices. Whether caregiving comes to you as the result of a health-care crisis or the progressive decline of the older adult, many choices and decisions have to be made—often very quickly. Most families are not prepared.They don't know what choices are available, what decisions are appropriate, and where to find needed resources. By completing this workbook before the first (or next) crisis arises, you can ease your decision-making process and reduce everyone's emotional stress.

Hard Questions, Simple Answers focuses on those life issues specific to older adults. Each section contains vital and necessary information, which will help you catalog the older adult's personal information, medical-insurance data, physical and mental status, legal and financial issues, the emotions of caregiving, the decision-making process, housing alternatives, and end-of-life issues. The appendices contain public and private resources, a glossary of caregiving terms, a bibliography, and articles that may assist you with solutions regarding an older adult's life issues.

As a social services professional and private geriatric care manager, I have assisted seniors, the frail elderly, and their families for twenty-eight years. This workbook was inspired by those caring, but frustrated family members who needed advice and counsel. They arrived in my office bearing files, stacks of papers, numerous post-it notes, and dozens of phone numbers, all of which only added to the overwhelming task of being a responsible adult child. This workbook simplified caregiving for them—and it can do the same for you.

Keep it accessible.

Good luck, and have faith in your abilities.

You are your older adult's best asset.

Elana Peters

Chapter One

The emotions of caregiving for you, the caregiver.

You're a caregiver! Caregiving to an older adult family member is different than any previous experience you may have had. For many, caregiving can bring the rich rewards of personal fulfillment and sharing love. Caring for an older adult can strengthen relationships and enhance life experiences. Caregiving can be the time in which differences can be reconciled and past grievances healed. You may have become a caregiver to keep a promise, while others of you may want to avoid the costs of assisted living. Caregiving may come naturally to you, but other family members may not want to share in the caregiving experience and may have to be coaxed into responding and cooperating. Each family, and each of its members, may have different motives for their response to caregiving opportunities.

What is the reason you are caregiving? It is important to evaluate your reason for caregiving as it will strongly effect the outcome you can expect from the experience. Are you caring for an older adult as a gift, or do you see it as your duty, or perhaps a debt to be repaid? You will either have a stressful experience that is full of negativity and resentment, or an experience of acceptance and peace depending on your motives.

Is your motive for caregiving a gift? If it's a gift, the burdens and responsibilities will be easier to bear. The older adult's physical and mental decline will be easier to accept, the frailties of their personality can often be met with humor, and the eventual outcome of their decline will be seen as a natural consequence of life. The gift of caregiving can bring feelings of satisfaction and encouragement. Along the way you may discover inner strength you did not realize you had and find a new inner peace to cope with the daily challenges. And when the caregiving time is over, you will feel a sense of gratitude for having had this privilege.

Caregivers who respond out of duty have a more difficult time coping with the negative emotions that come as a natural part of caregiving. If you feel as though you "have to do it" or "should do it," feelings of frustration, resentment, and anger will rise to the surface over and over again. These feelings are usually followed by guilt because you had them in the first place. You may ask yourself why you have to be the caregiver. This is especially true if you didn't have a good relationship with the older adult in your early years. The duty-filled caregiver suffers even more if abuse or abandonment was a part of the past. Although issues from the past may have been hidden or buried for many years, they will be remembered and become a part of the caregiving experience.

If your caregiving is seen as a debt to be repaid, you will be in a no-win situation. The older adult or parent may have brought you into this world and raised you to be a responsible adult, however there is no reasonable way that you can repay them for that. Raising a child and caring for an older adult are two very different situations—-as different as apples are from oranges. When one raises a child there are ages and stages of growth and development; there are goals and expectations as the child grows more and more independent. Childrearing experiences are passed down through the generations. If you want to improve this child-raising experience, you can read up on the latest theories of child development to change destructive patterns. Not so with older adults. There is no way to predict at what age a specific change in health or a social loss will occur. There are no clear stages for older adults. They are aging individuals who are vastly different from one another. These differences in the aging process vary widely and from individual to individual according to their personality, their ethnicity, their nationality, their life experiences, and their previous coping skills. For better or for worse, the older adult has peculiarities and frailties that are here to stay.

Whether by choice or default the caregiving role will not be, for many reasons, an easy task. Caregiving is a demanding, time consuming, energy-robbing experience that requires action, patience, planning, and flexibility. The difficult demands and hard work may be somewhat offset by the personal benefits received. You, as a caregiver, however, may reach a time when the demands will outweigh the benefits, especially if you find you are physically or emotionally exhausted. These stresses can negatively effect your health, attitude, relationships, career, and more. It can affect your ability to be the kind of caregiver you want to be, which adds to the exhaustion and stress.

If you are the primary caregiver, it makes you the family member or friend upon whom the older adult can depend. This means watching a once strong and capable adult decline into childlike behaviors and capabilities. This alone can be heartbreaking. Add to it an older adult's lack of cooperation and seeming ingratitude, then frustration and anger will become your companions. As the primary caregiver you are the one who will try to find and locate the best quality, most appropriate, and least expensive resources.

The older adult may insist that you not spend the money, but it will be necessary if they are to maintain their activities of daily living, while retaining as much of their independence as possible. It often means that you must become instrumental in making the older adult's care decisions or health choices even though the older adult resists and feels that they do not need yours or anyone's help.

Being the primary caregiver means you have assumed the responsibility for the older adult's well-being. You may even feel as though you are now in charge of their life, but you're not. This older adult, unless severely impaired mentally, needs to maintain as much choice in their care as possible and as much independence as their health will allow. Meanwhile, you may have to sit on the sidelines waiting for them to make decisions that are in their best interests. Underlying this resistance is their strong desire to remain independent, and not have anyone assist them. Their fear is that they will be seen as unable to care for themselves and will be forced to move out of their home.

You, the caregiver, may have to watch and wait for a crisis to happen before a decision for care can be made. Much too often this is the case, watching and waiting for an accident, a stroke, or a fall before you can get them the help they need. It's reasonable to feel anxious in this watch-and-wait situation.

You want to feel that the older adult is safe, reasonably comfortable, and is as content as possible under the circumstances. However, in many cases, the older adult may manipulate you into thinking that you have their cooperation, then an hour or a day later they may accuse you of treating them like a child or trying to put them away so you can take their money. They may not perceive your attempts at helping them as loving or caring. Is it any wonder that caregiving can be a seesaw of emotions?

The variety of emotions can run the gamut from loving tenderness to unbridled fury. Having negative emotions can make you feel guilty even though all of your emotions and feelings are real and normal. Many caregivers have had these feelings and they may go on for days, weeks, or months. Resentment may build because no one seems to understand the difficulties or offers to help you. As time passes you may begin to feel hopeless, which in turn makes you feel even worse, adding feelings of guilt. It's an exhausting and vicious circle.

What can you do to lessen the emotional cost of providing care? Accept from the beginning that you cannot be all things to the older adult. It is important to realize that you cannot make them well or happy. If they were never happy, or content, or easy to get along with, don't expect them to start now. If you are still trying to win their approval and praise, you will be disappointed.

Through the trials and errors of life, you have probably learned that love is not always nice, sweet, or perfect. Love is an action word, not just a noun, more than just a feeling. As an action, love involves considerable patience, endurance, and firmness. When adult children become primary caregivers, they have to be realistic in their assessment. Your older adult is still the same individual they always were, except now they are losing strength and energy. Struggling with maintaining their control and independence uses up much of the energy they had reserved for thoughtfulness, courtesy, and appreciation. So you will need to find the appreciation you deserve in other ways and from other sources: from family, friends, or support groups.

Setting limits

How truly sad it is that for many adult children, "To honor thy father and mother" has come to mean they have no right to honor themselves. Setting limits entails recognizing and accepting what you realistically can and cannot do for your older relatives, and then communicating this to them in an empathetic and sensitive manner. Setting limits is not an act of selfishness, but of caring for yourself so you can continue to care for them. More often than not, aging parents will surprise you, and accommodate your needs. Aging parents do not want to be alienated from their children; they have a need to be wanted and loved by them. When limits are set by the adult child based on knowing their personal strengths and weaknesses, rather than from anger, older adults usually respond positively.

Setting limits with aging parents is different from setting them for children. With children the limits are imposed on them. With older adults the limits are really based on you and your capacity not theirs. You can set limits on your caregiving time and efforts; set limits on your older adult's negative behaviors or verbal abuse. You may need to tell your frail, aging father or mother that their way of speaking to you is not acceptable, a difficult task for many people—after all, your parents brought you up not to talk back to them. Setting limits is imperative if you want to physically and emotionally survive the caregiving experience.

How do you determine what is a demand and what is a requirement? A requirement is a task or chore that will keep the older adult physically safe and as independent as their declining health will allow. It is based on a critical need given their physical or mental situation. A demand is a personal preference given by the older adult to the caregiver on how to meet a perceived requirement. By understanding the differences, you will be able to see more of the choices and options available in your caregiving situation.

The following may help you understand the difference between requirements and demands

- Evaluate the older adult's limitations and other resources that can help. If you find their requests burdensome, ask yourself how much of your help is actually needed.
- Consider the long-range effects on the older adult if you allow them to become unnecessarily dependent on you. Allowing them as much independence as possible is strongly related to their own sense of well-being.
- Accept your limitations. If you do too much, then burnout, who will be there to help when assistance is really needed?
- Respect the dignity of the older adult when you respond to their requests.
- Help them find and arrange for needed services, rather than doing it all for them.
- Agree to provide only those services you can manage gracefully and with good humor. Remember, when assistance is provided out of guilt, it creates feelings of frustration and anger.
- Stick to your decisions. If you consider a request unreasonable or unmanageable, explain your position and make alternative suggestions.
- Don't feel you have to continually justify yourself with the older adult or other family members.
- Realize you are not responsible for the older adult's happiness. Often people have trouble accepting the losses of old age, and they look for someone to blame for their distress. Accepting blame and feeling guilty about the older adult's dissatisfactions doesn't help either one of you.
- Let your parent know you care, even though you may not always meet all of their requests.
- Show your affection spontaneously by sharing special times, by touching, by hugging, by calling to share news or writing brief notes.

- Remember any change with an older adult takes patience, tenacity, and time.
- If you are having difficulty setting limits or saying, "no," join a support group where you'll find other caregivers who can offer suggestions, support and humor for your caregiving tasks.

If the older adult's behavior is jeopardizing their safety and well-being, it may be time for tough love. Tough love means taking a stand and setting limits. Tough love can be extremely difficult, especially when applied to a parent or beloved older relative. Tough love can bring with it feelings of discomfort and guilt. However, if you are going to survive, you must set limits with the older adult and with other family members as well.

Avoiding Caregiver Burnout

Although caregiving for an older adult can be rewarding, it can also be incredibly stressful. All too often family caregivers find that the stress outweighs the rewards of caregiving. The constancy of the day in and day out routine of caring for an older adult can be overwhelming and debilitating.

Sometimes the emotional stress of providing care tends to be greater than the physical or financial costs, since caregivers frequently give up personal renewal time. As a result of multiple responsibilities, caregiving can cause serious illness, depression, or even death to the caring family member. Known as caregiver burnout, it affects at least 44% of family caregivers. The good news is that there are things you can do to prevent burnout.

Even though a caregiver may think, "Why doesn't someone offer to help me?" or "How long will I have to do this? " They generally don't actually ask others for help nor do they seek out community resources. Family members may sacrifice a job, hobbies, leisure time, vacations, and/or privacy in order to caregive. When concerned people question these sacrifices or make suggestions to get help, a caregiver may reply, "Well, my parent (mother, father, grandparent) took care of me, now it's my turn to take care of them." That may be how you feel or what you believe, but as mentioned, taking care of an older adult is vastly different from caring for a child.

Instead of gratitude, a litany of complaints about what isn't right or what needs to be done, or detailed descriptions of their physical ailments may be the caregivers only feedback.

The idea of taking personal time is usually at the bottom of the caregiver's "to do" list. The health concerns and well-being of the older adult often depend on the ability of the caregiver to adroitly handle all of the details. Keeping track of multiple medications, doctors appointments, housekeeping, laundry, marketing, cooking, and the personal care needs of the older adult is almost an impossible task. Watching an older adult's memory and personality slip away due to dementia and then realize that the older adult is approaching the end of life, can be emotionally overwhelming. Having to face excessive physical demands as well as emotional demands makes you vulnerable to serious illness of your own, such as stroke, heart attack, depression, alcohol abuse, and abuse or neglect of the older adult.

Top five emotions of caregivers: Guilt, Frustration, Sadness, Resentment Anger. These are normal feelings!

Caregiving is not a job to be taken lightly, nor are the mood swings and emotional ups and downs to be ignored. Look over the following check-list. If you answer "yes" to any of them, you might be on the road to depression and burnout:

Warning Signs of Stress/Depression:

Yes	No	
___	___	Difficulty falling asleep or remaining asleep.
___	___	Waking up early, feeling anxious and irritable
___	___	Marked changes in appetite/weight
___	___	Increased use of sleeping pills, alcohol or other medications

Yes	No	
___	___	Uncharacteristic short-temperedness, crying or agitation
___	___	Neglect of physical/hygiene needs
___	___	Loss of energy or fatigue
___	___	Subdued mood—flat voice, expressionless face
___	___	Rough handling and other signs of impatience in giving care
___	___	Recurrent thoughts of death or suicide

THREE BEST WAYS to Set Limits

1. Know and accept your limitations
2. Offer parents alternatives before saying "NO"
3. In a kind way, let them know what behaviors are not tolerable.

Are you making time for:

Yes	No	
___	___	Personal renewal: doing what you truly enjoy
___	___	Exercise: Walking, jogging, swimming, etc.
___	___	Recreation: a movie, a visit with friends, time with family
___	___	Quiet time: spiritual, meditation, visualization
___	___	Humor: laugh at a joke, play with your kids or grandkids

You, as a caregiver, need respite in this demanding role. Taking personal respite is a way to re-energize. Making the time and taking it, even if only for a half-hour daily, offers a calmer perspective and way to revitalize that sense of self. Making time for a walk in the neighborhood, lunch with a good friend, a manicure, a movie, or watching a grandchild's soccer game is great respite. If you do not make time for respite, then you might become the one who needs full time care.

In addition to taking time for yourself, you need to review your role as caregiver. Are you doing too much, without any time for yourself? Is there a way you can make it easier or more organized? Review the following list to help you get back on track. It may be easier than you think.

1. Accept that "trying to do it all' is usually an impossible task. Take a realistic look by making a checklist of all that is to be done, including your own family's needs and obligation. Are you surprised, that it sounds like a job for Superwoman?
2. Think of the activities you miss the most. Begin to plan for at least one of them within the next two weeks. Make a contract with yourself, by setting the date, the activity, and then doing it.
3. Connect with a local program or service that will allow for an hour or two of worry-free respite. There are many agencies or programs available in the community. The local senior center, the Area Agency on Aging, the Alzheimer's Association, all offer good information that can assist in locating appropriate resources and assistance, such as in-home help, overnight care, adult day care, and support groups.

Yes, if you look there is help out there even though it may take several telephone calls or inquiries of friends. It is most important that you have some rest and renewal and time away from the older adult. Self-care is not an act of selfishness, it is intrinsically connected with effectively providing care to the older adult. Self-care will make your job less stressful and make it easier to cope with the changes in the older adult and enhance the quality of your caregiving tasks.

The emotions of being cared for: The older adult

As natural as aging is, it's a subject that most individuals do not want to think or talk about.Talking about aging is personally uncomfortable and socially awkward. All aspects of aging seem fearful, from loss of looks to loss of health. In an attempt to keep the inevitable at a safe distance, Americans spend millions of dollars annually on vitamins, diet fads, creams, and cosmetic surgery.

The dichotomy of aging is that many who reach the advanced age of eighty, ninety, or one hundred years, are proud of this accomplishment. However, many of these elders think of their longevity as entitlement, and set unrealistic expectations on their adult children. They conveniently forget that these adult children are in mid-life with numerous responsibilities, such as their own family.

With age the body does become more vulnerable to illness and disease. This is normal, denying or ignoring the aging process does not reverse it or make it go away. More often than not, living to "a ripe old age" means needing assistance in managing one's daily life to remain as independent as long as possible.The reality is that eighty percent of older adults past eighty years of age have one or more chronic illnesses that may limit activities of daily living, such as cooking, cleaning, shopping, driving, bathing and dressing. To deny this reality is foolish and makes it difficult for everyone concerned—the elder, the adult children, the paid care provider, or the administrative staff in an assisted living environment.

And yet knowing this, many elders insist that only an adult child can be "the care provider." While others expect their adult children to carry the sole burden of responsibility for making them feel less lonely and isolated. These elders often demand, manipulate, and push all of the guilt buttons in order to have their way.

An older adult or aging parent wants to be nurtured and feel loved at this time in life, yet many make it next to impossible to love them, let alone want to be in their company. Discontent with this twilight time there are endless

FIVE TOP INDICATORS of Caregiver Burnout

1. Feelings of helplessness or hopelessness.
2. Gain or loss of weight.
3. Changes in health or difficulty recovering from colds/flu.
4. Increased intake in amounts of alcohol, prescription drugs or over-the-counter medications.
5. Lashing out, physically or verbally toward the older adult.

complaints, a litany of past mistakes, nit-picky criticisms, and chronic ingratitude, all adding up to an older adult who makes life difficult for themselves and for those that care about them.

For many older adults, the expectations of life's Golden Years far outweigh the realities of what adult children or family can provide physically, financially, and, most of all, emotionally. These aging individuals have endured the Great Depression, the trauma of World War II, and witnessed the pain, suffering, and early loss of loved ones because medical science had not yet made its phenomenal advances. These older individuals were focused on basic needs and survival. So for many of them learning to count their blessings, expressing their gratitude, or being happy was never a priority.

FIVE BEST WAYS of an Aging Adult: Loneliness, Abandonment, Loss of independence, Concern about running out of money, Having to move from their home.

A closer examination of the older adult's life may reveal a frightened individual, whose health is declining and now requiring assistance from others. Losing independence is not easy for those who have survived many losses and are in the midst of experiencing others—the loss of a spouse, close friends, a pet, home, and/or health can occur in rapid succession. Accompanying these losses are often feelings of loneliness, isolation, or abandonment, all normal parts of being human. Many older adults, experiencing these losses, expect the adult child to step in and fill the gaps, to make them feel better and possibly take away both the physical and emotional pain.

Is it fair to expect so much from an adult child? Can an adult child become the hands-on caregiver as well as be the provider of the older individual's emotional needs? These older adults often overlook the fact that the other adult is aging, too. They still see these busy mid-life adults as their children and expect them to be available, often on a moment's notice, to run errands, go to the doctor, provide physical assistance, in addition to making them happy.

Adult children may be able to improve the older adult's life, but make them happy? NO WAY! Most information about caring for aging individuals focuses on teaching the adult child how to cope with the disagreeable behaviors of the older adult. Informational materials for aging adults that offer suggestions on how to age graciously, grow old in wisdom and love, and show appreciation for today's blessings are lacking.

To fill this gap, the following guidelines are offered to the aging individual on behalf of their adult children:

- Honor your adult children. Love them because you are lucky to have them.
- Make your adult children feel appreciated, not guilty. Offer praise freely.
- Do as much as possible for yourself; your adult children have many responsibilities and demands on their time. They are aging, too!
- Keep your sense of humor. Make your adult child glad to be sharing time with you.
- Learn the difference between sharing and complaining.
- Keep your adult children informed about what is happening to you and be as objective as possible.
- Let your adult children help you stay in charge of your life. Be loving but firm about making your own decisions, based on reasonable choices.
- Accept your growing dependence, that is a part of the aging process.
- Seek out alternative resources that offer assistance before you need them. This will give your adult children peace of mind.
- Your adult child does not know how to be old or how to accept death. Teach them with your wisdom and experience.
- Be considerate of your adult children's time and assistance, so they won't become exhausted, resentful, and burned out.
- Remember that a concerned and caring adult child is an aging adult's best asset.

The best you can do for the older adult is to empower them and help them retain their independence as long as possible. The worst is to move into their lives and take over everything. The less you can do for your older relative (depending on physical and mental abilities) the better it is for everyone. What ever is done must be done with the older adult, and not for them.

The key to successfully managing the tasks involved with caregiving is to allow the older adult as much control over their lives and decisions as possible. Remember to ask them what they want, don't tell them what is best for them.This temptation can be extremely difficult to overcome. Sometimes all you may be able to do is offer suggestions and not make their choices. Perhaps you may need to remind them of the possible consequences of their not following through with these suggestions.

Often all you can do is to remind yourself that you are doing your best under the circumstances. Then let go, you may be pleasantly surprised at the outcome.

Chapter Two

Collecting the older adult's essential financial, legal and medical information.

If you feel as though your life, the older adult's life, and things in general are out of control, getting the necessary basic personal information together will help immensely. This is the information that will serve you long and well if you can gain control over it now. Organizing the information will clarify many issues and help make your caregiving responsibilities run smoother.

As you know, today's health care system is complex and vastly different from what it was like even a few years ago. Technology has assisted in extending life expectancy, but it has also created a complex system of communication. Everything seems to move more quickly now. Older adults, who have chronic illnesses and are in declining health, often have difficulty with these newer systems. Family members must have the ability to help their older relatives maneuver through these new health care systems.

Make several copies of the personal information & medical insurance data. You will be asked for them over and over.

There are three basic areas of focus that can assist you in making progress through the current health care system: personal, financial, and legal. This section organizes the basic information you will need to have on hand when applying for private or public assistance, when admitting the older adult into a hospital, an emergency room, or a health care or alternative living arrangement. By gathering and organizing this kind of information you will learn what to plan for in the caregiving tasks ahead. Most importantly, being organized now will allow you to more efficiently utilize the available resources to benefit the well-being of the older adult when a crisis occurs.

At this point you may think that you need to involve the family in the care planning. In reality, it is better to wait until you clearly understand what you want to achieve on behalf of the older adult before involving everyone. To do this you must obtain the information on the following pages and have a pre-plan before you involve other family members in a caregiving discussion. If you do not, you may get knocked off course by their suggestions and opinions.

Basic personal information

This section has two critical parts: personal information and the medical insurance data of the older adult.

The following basic personal information about the older adult can be filled out, then copied so that you can take it with you to the various service providers, community resources, and health care facilities. This information, gathered together and completed, will help you both feel as though you have accomplished an important task. Although this is only one of the many known and unknown tasks that may lie ahead, completing this one will bring some relief from at least part of the stress.

Personal Information sheet

Name ______________________________

Maiden name______________ Nickname ______________

Address ______________________________

City ______________ State ________ Zip ________

Phone ( ) __________ FAX __________ email __________

Social security # ____-____-____ Medicare # ______________

Driver's License __________ Other vital #s __________

DOB ______________ Age ________ Sex ________

Place of Birth ______________________________

Marital Status ___ Married __ Widowed __ Divorced __ Single __

Separated ___

For how long? ______________________________

Name of spouse ______________________ Age ________

Social Security # ____-____-____ Driver's license ______________

Does the spouse live with the older adult who needs assistance?

___ Yes ___ No

Spouse's health problems and concerns ______________

____

Medical insurance data

Fill out the Medical Insurance Data accurately. This information determines eligibility for many benefits and is required in every health care situation. The same questions will be asked frequently, so keep this information handy.

Any adult, 65 years or older, is usually eligible for Medicare, the federal government's health care reimbursement program. However, Medicare requires deductibles and a monthly premium and does not pay for prescription medications or custodial care. A supplemental health care policy (aka MediGap) is usually needed for more complete health care coverage.

Many older adults who are eligible for Medicare join Health Maintenance Organizations (HMO) because they require minimal deductibles and offer many prescriptions drugs as part of the coverage. If your older adult is a member of an HMO, they will not need a MediGap policy because the HMO assumes the health care risk of the enrollee. The federal health care agency pays a specific amount in the name of the enrollee to the HMO on a monthly basis. Even if the older adult does not use any benefits, the HMO still gets paid.

If your older adult has joined an HMO, your advocacy for good health care coverage is mandatory

To date, HMOs have not provided the same kind of old-fashioned health care that is familiar to this generation of older adults. They grew up in the years when physicians were looked upon as infallible. Today's complex, specialist-oriented system can be extremely frustrating for them, not to mention detrimental to their health and well-being.

If you or the older adult find yourselves frustrated with the quality of health care provided, call the Customer Relations Department of the HMO and complain loudly and persistently. If the results do not meet your satisfaction, call the nearest Health Insurance Counseling Advocacy Program (HICAP) office. They will assist and guide you on what to do next and the service is free. You can also call HICAP before speaking to your HMO's customer relations department.

Upon request, they will mail out unbiased comparison lists of HMOs, MediGap Policies, and Long-Term Care Insurance Policies that will give you a clearer understanding of the benefits each provides.

Medical insurance information

Does the older adult have medical insurance? _____ Yes ______ No

❑ **Medicare**

Medicare # _______________ Part A ______ Part B _____

❑ **MediGap policy**

Name of insurance ___________________________ Group #____________

Policy agent ____________________________ Phone __________________

❑ **HMO**

Name of HMO ____

Membership # _________________________________

Affiliate name __________________________ Phone __________________

❑ **Long Term Care (LTC) policy**

Policy name _________________________________

Policy # ____________________________________

Agent ________________ Phone __________________

Do the LTC benefits cover...

Nursing home care ____ Residential care ____ In-Home care ______

Deductible period __________ Daily benefit ______________

Length of coverage __________________________________

❑ **SSI**

Case number __________________

Case/ social worker ______________ Phone ____________________

❑ **Medi-Cal**

Case number ___________________

Case/ social worker _______________ Phone __________

❑ **Durable power of attorney for health care (DPAHC)**

Yes ____ No ____ When was it last updated? __________

Be specific about: Hydration ____ Feeding Tubes ____ Iffs ____

Antibiotics ____ Resuscitation ____ Other life-sustaining measures

____

Basic financial information

More time can be spent caring for an elderly parent than in raising a child—lasting from 1 to 20 years. Yet most family members wait until there is a crisis, then seek out services to care for the older adult. This is when the adult children find that the finances or the health insurance requirements, or the elder's manipulative threats of disinheritance or ending one's life, a major detriment to making a sane decision. Hasty or incorrect choices are often made at this critical time, which can bankrupt a family not only financially, but emotionally.

Make at least 6 copies of the DPAHC. Give copies to physicians, hospitals, home-care staff, care facilities, etc. Keep a copy in the primary caregiver's file and another one visibly accessible in the elder's home.

In general, older adults want to preserve their accumulated savings and assets "just in case." They think "it"—that is, becoming incapacitated and dependent on others—is not going to happen to them. Most have not given much thought to their future because they did not plan on requiring any assistance. And, even when they are facing a health decline and suffering physical setbacks, they do not want to spend their money. So having a discussion about money and fiscal issues with an older adult may not be an easy task and yet it is imperative to do so.

The following basic financial information about the older adult can be filled out, then copied so that it will be available when seeking public or private assistance, community resources, or when considering alternative living arrangements. Today's resources are not "cheap," therefore this information will give you a realistic picture of what kind of care the older adult can afford.

Although many older adults find it difficult to discuss finances with their children or other relatives, it is vitally important they do so. If the older adult becomes incapacitated and their financial status is not known, the family can face costly legal fees or long delays establishing conservatorship, unless their children can have access to this information.

Personal Income

Monthly Income

Income Sources

Social Security $ ____________________

Pension $ ____________________

Veterans Benefits $ ____________________

SS Disability $ ____________________

Public Assistance/SSI $ ____________________

Other $ ____________________

Real Property $ ____________________

Where does the older adult live?

Own home ___ Condo ___ Mobile home ___ Apartment ___ Other ___

Address ____

City ____________________________ State ____ Zip ________________

Purchase Price $__________________________

Approximate value of owned home $ _________________________________

Is there a Mortgage(s) Yes ___ No ___

Value $ ____________________

Financial Estate

Approximate Cash on-hand: $ ____________________

Bank Accounts $ ____________________

Institution ____

Type ____

Branch ____

Phone ______________________________

Account# __________________________

Amount $ ___________________

Institution ____

Type ____

Branch ____

Phone ______________________________

Account# __________________________

Amount $ ___________________

Institution ____

Type ____

Branch ____

Phone ______________________________

Account# __________________________

Amount $ ___________________

Additional Financial Assets

Any Additional Real Property? Yes ___ No ___

Approximate value $ ____________________

Purchase Price $ ____________________

Mortgage $ ____________________

Address ____

City ____________________________ State ____ Zip ________________

Jewelry $ ____________________

Antiques $ ____________________

Other valuables $ ____________________

Type ____

____

Does the older adult own a car? Yes ___ No ___

Approximate value $ ____________________

License number _____________________

Make _____________________ Model _____________________

Is registration current? Yes ___ No ___

Expiration date _____________________

Currently drive? Yes ___ No ___

If no, explain ____

____

Stocks and Bonds

Company ______________________________ Phone _________________________

Number of Shares ____________________

Purchase Cost $ ______________________

Current Value $ ______________________

Broker ____

Company ______________________________ Phone _________________________

Number of Shares ____________________

Purchase Cost $ ______________________

Current Value $ ______________________

Broker ____

Company ______________________________ Phone _________________________

Number of Shares ____________________

Purchase Cost $ ______________________

Current Value $ ______________________

Broker ____

Life Insurance

Company ______________________________ Phone _________________________

Policy ____________________________________

Insured ____

Benefit $ ____________________

Face Value $ ____________________

Beneficiary(ies) ____

____

Liabilities/Creditors

Company ________________________ Phone ____________________

Amount Due $ ____________________

Interest Rate ____________________ Due Date ____________________

Company ________________________ Phone ____________________

Amount Due $ ____________________

Interest Rate ____________________ Due Date ____________________

Company ________________________ Phone ____________________

Amount Due $ ____________________

Interest Rate ____________________ Due Date ____________________

Company ________________________ Phone ____________________

Amount Due $ ____________________

Interest Rate ____________________ Due Date ____________________

Company ________________________ Phone ____________________

Amount Due $ ____________________

Interest Rate ____________________ Due Date ____________________

Basic legal information

Older adults who do not have their legal affairs in order before a health care crisis or long-term illness, may impoverish themselves as well as depleting the physical and emotional reserves of family members. If the older adult becomes unable to handle their own affairs and has not completed the necessary legal documents and/or made appropriate arrangements, then court actions, such a guardianships or conservatorships, may be initiated in their interest. These legal actions are expensive and humiliating.

Many older adults, for various reasons, are not always able to understand the legal issues and the importance of seeking the professional advice of an attorney. One of the best gifts an older adult can give to their family is to plan ahead, and discuss all fiscal issues and legal aspects of long-term care with an attorney or other trusted individual before the need arises. There is a relatively new specialty in the practice of law called elder law, which can assist older adults and family members with their legal issues and concerns. The cost is well worth the peace of mind you will receive if you use an elder law attorney.

The following basic legal information about the older adult can be filled out and taken with you to the attorney, or when applying for public or private assistance. This information is of the utmost importance if you want to preserve the older adult's assets in order to better provide for their care.

Legal information sheet

Gather all of the following papers, documents, and data in one place, checking to see if the professional advisors are current and the documents are up to date and/or still valid.

Important articles	Location
Safety deposit key	______________________
Bank account information	______________________
Health insurance policy	______________________
Social Security card	______________________
Medicare/health insurance cards	______________________

Important articles	**Location**
Life insurance policy	______________
Home or property deed of sale	______________
Will	______________
Living trust (if applicable)	______________
Living will (or medical directive)	______________
Power of attorney	______________
Income tax returns	______________
Pre-paid burial plot or vault receipt	______________
Funeral instructions	______________
Birth certificate	______________
Marriage license	______________
Divorce papers	______________
Important contracts	______________
Mortgages	______________
Credit card accounts	______________
Inventory of personal property	______________

Professional Advistors

Attorney ______________ Phone ______________

Attorney ______________ Phone ______________

Accountant ______________ Phone ______________

Insurance Agent ______________ Phone ______________

Insurance Agent ______________________ Phone ______________________

Stockbroker _________________________ Phone ______________________

Financial Planner _____________________ Phone ______________________

Bank/Trust Officer ___________________ Phone ______________________

Clergyman __________________________ Phone ______________________

Executor/Trustee ____________________ Phone ______________________

Address ____

City ___________________________ State _________ Zip ________________

Phone _________________________ Fax ___________________

Health Care Agent ____

Address ____

City ___________________________ State _________ Zip ________________

Phone _________________________ Fax ___________________

Is there a Do Not Resuscitate (DNR) Order? Yes ___ No ___

If Yes, notify all home caregivers of the DNR and place in a conspicuous place

DO NOT CALL 911

CALL THE LOCAL HOSPITAL EMERGENCY ROOM

PHONE ________________

Chapter Three

Recruiting the family to help.

Now you are going to focus on a different kind of information. This kind of information is going to require you to be realistic and to become familiar with the reliability and talents of your family members. This information does not exist on paper anywhere. You must create and collect this information in order to provide better assistance, receive valuable input, and more efficiently manage the older adult's caregiving situation.

The Primary Caregiver

If you are reading this book, you are probably the primary caregiver. As the primary caregiver you are the family member who will take responsibility for making the critical health, caregiving, and organizational decisions on behalf of the older adult. Before committing to this role, realistically look at your time limitations due to other responsibilities such as a spouse, children, and/or work. AND, this is the big one, you must take responsibility for yourself, so you will be sure to make time for respite and recreation.

This primary caregiver role is established early on in life; it is the family member who can take charge of a situation and get the job done. Each and every family has one. The primary caregiver can be a son, yet 75 percent of the time it is a daughter. The one to become the primary caregiver is usually closest to the older adult emotionally or geographically. As the primary caregiver you are going to manage this job differently from any other task, job, or position you may have had previously.

At first you may think that you can handle all of the tasks by yourself because no one else can do the job quite like you can. However, you will quickly learn that this management position can become overwhelming, burdensome, and lonely, if not shared with others. You will need to call upon your siblings or other family members to assist you with this care. If you are an only child or cannot secure the help of family members, then you will need to seek resources in the community to assist you with the older adult's care. Alone, you cannot succeed.

As the primary caregiver you need to meet and discuss with other family members the seriousness of the caregiving responsibilities. The purpose of this discussion is, hopefully, to have each and every family member come to the same level of mutual understanding regarding the level of care the older adult needs now and may need in the future. Then you can establish which sibling or family member can help you with the necessary and particular caregiving tasks or chores. Remember, assign only those tasks to those individuals that will make a commitment and have the required talent.

Top five statements of older adults when talking to their adult children about money.

1. Can't we find someone cheaper?

2. Why can't you (adult child) help me out?

3. You only want to spend my money.

4. You want to put me away.

5. I am saving it as your inheritance.

At this point, you may be wondering what talents you or your family members have. This is not about being an artist, a sculptor or a writer. A talent, for the purposes of caregiving, is a particular ability or skill that a sibling, relative, friend, or neighbor may be able to contribute to ease problems or save money. These talents will be able to assist with the many tasks and chores you may be called upon to contribute to the caregiving situation. Some talents include: bill paying, bookkeeping, cooking, cleaning, driving, staying overnight, visiting, going on doctor visits, financial assistance, coupons, groceries, laundry, shopping, medication management, home maintenance, gardening, mowing the lawn, putting out the trash, painting, appliance repair, telephoning, providing home cooked meals that can be frozen. As you plan and look at your options for care of the older adult, review everyone's availability for providing assistance. What talent will each individual be able to contribute?

Some family members will respond graciously, others will be available only occasionally, others will reluctantly agree, and others will decline. Each and every one, however, needs to contribute something, in some cases it may be money or only a weekly telephone call. Always accept even the smallest contribution with appreciation, you will be glad you did!

You will need to ask each and every family member what they can contribute to assist you. Be very specific about what talents are needed, and when they offer, assign them the chore or task.Then get a commitment for time and place. Let them know that the older adult is relying on them to be there at that time and on that day. It is extremely important that they understand the value of what they are contributing. Sometimes family members need to have what they are doing translated into dollars and cents. Tell them that what they are contributing with their time and talents is saving money and they are contributing to the caregiving situation to help make it work.

Before you ask assistance and assign specific tasks, you will need to realistically assess your older adult's caregiving needs. You will need to evaluate the kind and type of care the older adult will need to remain as independent and as comfortable as possible. Establishing financial feasibility is an important factor to discuss with other family members and the older adult

It is important at this stage that you begin to communicate with the older adult and with other family members about the needs of the older adult. The caregiving process may be very new to everyone involved. It may take time for some people, especially the older adult, to come to terms with the changes that lie ahead. Often the first objective in your caregiving situation is simply to recognize that help is needed and that people are preparing to fill the needs.

When involving other family members clarity is crucial. Create a simple chart to organize the list of needs of the older adult.

TASKS	Daily	Weekly	Monthly	Periodic
Cooking				
Cleaning				
Driving				
Paying bills				
Telephoning				
Shopping				
Errands				
Visiting				
Gardening				
Maintenance				
Vacuuming				
Laundry				
Medication				

There are a variety of resources and services available in the community, some are free, some low cost and some costly. So establishing financial feasibility is an important factor to establish, and to discuss with other family members and the older adult.

Primary Caregiver form

Name ______________________________

Age ________________

Home Phone ________________ Work Phone________________

Address ____

City ________________________________ State ________ Zip _________

Relationship ________________________

Phone __________________________ Fax __________________________

Employed? Yes ___ No ___

Occupation____

Full Time ___ Part Time ___

Number of hours per week _________

Employer Name ____

Address ____

City ________________________________ State ________ Zip _________

Phone __________________________ Fax __________________________

Personal support system

Family members

Name ________________________________ Age ______

Address ______________________________________

Home phone ______________ Work phone ______________

FAX ________________ Email ______________________

Talent ______________ Availability ________________

Name ________________________________ Age ______

Address ______________________________________

Home phone ______________ Work phone ______________

FAX ________________ Email ______________________

Talent ______________ Availability ________________

Name ________________________________ Age ______

Address ______________________________________

Home phone ______________ Work phone ______________

FAX ________________ Email ______________________

Talent ______________ Availability ________________

Name ________________________________ Age ______

Address ____

Home phone _______________ Work phone _______________

FAX ____________________ Email ________________________

Talent _________________ Availability ___________________

What is a talent? Bookkeeping, bill paying, cooking, cleaning, dusting, taking over finances, driving, doctor's appointments, groceries, errands, shopping, staying overnight, visiting, offering respite to the primary care-giver,, telephoning, medication, management.

Additional relatives & extended family

Grandchildren, siblings, nieces, nephews, extended family and others who could offer assistance:

Name ____________________________________ Age ________

Address ____

Home phone _______________ Work phone _______________

FAX ____________________ Email ________________________

Talent _________________ Availability ___________________

Name ____________________________________ Age ________

Address ____

Home phone _______________ Work phone _______________

FAX ____________________ Email ________________________

Talent _________________ Availability ___________________

Name ____________________________________ Age ________

Address ____

Home phone _______________ Work phone _______________

FAX ____________________ Email ________________________

Talent _________________ Availability ___________________

Name ______________________________ Age ________

Address ____

Home phone ______________ Work phone ________________

FAX __________________ Email ________________________

Talent ________________ Availability ____________________

Name ______________________________ Age ________

Address ____

Home phone ______________ Work phone ________________

FAX __________________ Email ________________________

Talent ________________ Availability ____________________

Name ______________________________ Age ________

Address ____

Home phone ______________ Work phone ________________

FAX __________________ Email ________________________

Talent ________________ Availability ____________________

Name ______________________________ Age ________

Address ____

Home phone ______________ Work phone ________________

FAX __________________ Email ________________________

Talent ________________ Availability ____________________

Name ______________________________________ Age ________

Address ____

Home phone _______________ Work phone __________________

FAX ____________________ Email __________________________

Talent __________________ Availability ____________________

Name ______________________________________ Age ________

Address ____

Home phone _______________ Work phone __________________

FAX ____________________ Email __________________________

Talent __________________ Availability ____________________

Chapter Four

Assessing the older adult's physical needs.

This is the phase of caregiving where you must learn how to collect and organize subjective information. Although this is not an easy task, it can and must be done if you want to help the older adult. The difficult part of this phase is that the information you collect may change as the older adult becomes weaker or stronger. Therefore, the information that you collect now will need to be updated regularly so that you will be able to stay on top of any changes that may be taking place in the older adult's health and behaviors. By doing this you will be ready to make the wisest choice for care should the present situation no longer be appropriate. Always keep in mind that change is an integral and unavoidable part of the caregiving process.

Five reasonable objectives for caregivers of older adults: Safety, comfort, best care possible, loving attitude and peace of mind

Being able to assess an older adult's needs is a primary function in providing care to an older adult. The various tasks involved in caregiving will require you to make many choices and decisions that will be based on both objective and subjective information. There may be times when these decisions are clear cut, such as the scheduling of doctor visits, refills for prescriptions, or confirming the amount of money in the older adult's bank accounts.

There will be other times, however, when important decisions will be based on subjective information, that is, how you perceive the situation based on the best interests and safety of the older adult. This is when you need to realistically assess the older adults needs based on their current physical and mental status. Often, primary caregivers, siblings and other close relatives have difficulty "seeing" the older adult as they are: frail, failing, and with heightened personality quirks. Whether the wake-up call happens slowly or suddenly, it can be an emotional shock to all concerned and difficult to accept. Simultaneously, the older adult may be having difficulty coping with their own health changes and reluctant to give up any of their independence.

Because there may be conflicting opinions held among the primary caregiver, siblings and others involved, emotions can be on edge. This is the time and phase of caring when the assessment of the older adult should be seen as a vitally important necessary step toward successful caregiving.

You should recognize that as time goes by, things will naturally change. Although the older adult may have the ability to cope and perform the many activities of daily living today, that could change overnight. Being observant and aware of the possibility and probability of changes in the older adult's physical and mental status, and behaviors will help you in making the most appropriate decisions and choosing your options wisely.

Your adeptness at collecting the subjective information will help you, the various family members, and the many health providers involved, to more accurately assess the condition of the older adult and then recommend the most appropriate care for the current situation. The results of collecting the most accurate information will make the results of caregiving decisions more beneficial to the older adult and will simplify your caregiving tasks.

Assessing physical status

This section will assist you in providing an assessment of your older adult's physical capabilities and needs. Although your observations may be subjective, it is very important for you, the primary caregiver, to identify them to the best of your ability. Sometimes the older adult will try to cover up for their failings by changing the subject or confabulating information. If this seems to be happening, be patient and kind. If necessary, stop the probing and come back to it later. However, do not give up, be tenacious. This assessment step is crucial in the caregiving process.

Too often a large gap exists between the real needs of the older adult and their needs as perceived by the adult children. As an example, adult children may be overly concerned with the cleanliness of the home, laundry, or personal hygiene. From the older adult's point of view these concerns may be thought of as low priorities. Instead, the older adult's concerns may be with crime and safety in a deteriorating neighborhood, the difficulties of finding accurate information from a governmental agency, or just finding the energy to cope with daily living.

If you or other siblings have not spent much time in recent weeks or months being with and observing the older adult, you may not realize that their health needs have changed. The health changes are even more of a shock when adult children live a distance away and come to visit. You and others may not like seeing that the older adult's health is failing, making it even more difficult to accept that their safety and well-being is at risk. That is the reasoning behind the assessment tool enclosed in this chapter to enable you the primary caregiver "to see" the older adult in a more realistic light.

This assessment tool is a helpful checklist for you to use to establish the essential needs of the older adult. It is also a way of showing the other concerned adults who may involved, but are in doubt, that indeed the time has come where the older adult will need additional help and support with their personal care and the activities of daily living.

Sometimes you may have to ask the older adult how they manage certain tasks, and then subjectively assess them. Each level has certain criteria. As an example, can the older adult remember to take the necessary medications at the scheduled time? Are they able to set them out? Could they take their medications independently if they had a weekly pill reminder box that you set up for them? When different medications are taken at various hours of the day, you need to know that the older adult is able to manage their medication schedule and won't become confused or overwhelmed. When confused about medication time or dosage, an older adult may mistakenly think that it is okay to take their pills an hour earlier or an hour later, or if they forget one dose they may double the dose the next time.

Other examples of their capacity to accomplish ordinary activities are ones that may involve the older adult's ability to get in and out of a bathtub independently and safely. Are they having incontinence mishaps? Has being able to get on and off the toilet contributed to these mishaps? Has walking in and around their home become tedious and difficult for them. If they are off balance due to certain medications, they may need to have grab bars or safety rails installed in the bathrooms, hallways, or near their favorite chair or by the bed. Ramps can be installed over the small steps going in and out of the home. However, two story homes or apartments will be difficult for the older adult to manage and therefore are considered a safety hazard.

There are two separate categories of activities that measure the older adult's ability to live independently without assistance from another. The first category of activities is called Instrumental Activities of Daily Living also known in medical and insurance jargon as IADLs. These activities include cooking, laundry, housekeeping, driving, telephoning, and money management. Just because the older adult is unable to perform one or more of these activities doesn't mean they can't live alone. Needing help with these IADLs does not mean the older adult is incompetent; help with these activities are commonly available for individuals of all ages. Hiring one or more of these services may enable the older adult to live independently and maintain control of their daily life for a longer period of time.

The second category of activities is the warning indicators that the older adult is in a cautionary stage and is probably declining to the point where they will need hands-on care. Medical professionals and insurance companies call these Activities of Daily Living (ADLs) and the older adult is rated according to the level at which they are able to perform each of these required functions. These activities include eating, walking, bathing, dressing, grooming, toileting and incontinence. The ability to perform and complete these activities without help from another, whether a family member or paid care provider, is fundamental to an older adult's being able to live alone without assistance. If the older adult is unable to manage these activities alone but tells you they can, then they are jeopardizing their health and safety. Quite often, an older adult will neglect personal hygiene because they are no longer able to do it themselves. Unpleasant body odors are usually indicators that the older adult is neglecting personal hygiene and needs hands-on personal assistance. These activities of daily living can be provided by you, the primary caregiver, other family members, a paid care provider, by a home care agency, or at an assisted living facility.

If the older adult is able to perform all of these activities of daily living at a totally independent level, then living alone is considered still safe. If the older adult is able to perform these activities slowly but surely, then you need to be on alert as they will probably require some hands on assistance in the very near future. Once the older adult begins to be challenged in performing their household chores and/or personal hygiene routine, you need to discuss and plan how these activities can be accomplished in a reliable and safe manner. A fall, or a broken bone or hip, is all it takes for your life and the older adult's life to suddenly change before your eyes.

The information collected on these pages will be of vital use to everyone involved in the health and physical care of the older adult. Physicians and other professional health care providers must have a description of the older adult's capabilities with both Instrumental Activities of Daily Living (IADLs) and Activities of Daily Living (ADLs).

Five universal haunting issues for caregivers:

1. making the wrong decision,

2. something might happen to them if I am not the one providing the care

3. they could die in their home alone,

4. I am responsible for their happiness,

5. having to put them "someplace."

Primary physicians and other physicians involved in the older adult's care

The first step in assessing the older adult's physical status is to list the names and phone numbers of the primary physician and all other physician specialists that may have treated the older adult within the past two years. The physician's office nurse practitioner or the physician's nurse can answer many medical questions. If available, list those names, too.

Physicians

Physician ____________________ Specialty ______________________

Address ____

Phone _________________________ FAX _________________________

Date of last visit __________ Diagnosis _________________________

Physician is on staff at the following hospitals ____________________

____

Date of last visit ___________ Diagnosis ________________________

____

Does the primary physician's office have a nurse practitioner?

If so, what is her/his name? __________________

Other physicians involved in the older adult's care

Physician ____________________ Specialty ____________

Address ____

Phone _________________________ FAX _________________________

Date of last visit _________ Diagnosis __________________________

____

Physician ____________________ Specialty ____________

Address ____

Phone _________________________ FAX _________________________

Date of last visit __________ Diagnosis _________________________

____

Physician ____________________ Specialty ____________

Address ____

Phone _________________________ FAX __________________________

Date of last visit _________ Diagnosis __________________________

____

Physician ____________________ Specialty ____________

Address ____

Phone _________________________ FAX __________________________

Date of last visit _________ Diagnosis __________________________

____

Optimizing medical care for older adults

Many older adults find the current health care system overwhelming and complex. Too many of today's physicians tend to minimize concerns and over medicate for physical complaints. Older adult's who suffer from chronic illnesses or complex health problems need an advocate to ensure that they receive the best care from their physician or HMO. This advocate needs to a concerned and responsible adult and is usually the primary caregiver. The advocate makes sure that the older adult receives the appropriate treatment or services, if necessary, seeks to change or expand treatment to meet the older adult's needs, and may even intervene to make the current system more responsive.

It is of utmost importance that the physician fully grasps what is bothering the older adult. This may mean that the older adult (or their advocate) speaks up promptly, compellingly and even knowledgeably to get the required attention. To do this, the advocate may have to read about or research the health care problem and its current treatment(s). Questions may need to be asked, if the physician's explanations or instructions are unclear to you. You may need to bring up problems even if the physician doesn't ask, or tell them when a treatment or medication isn't having the desired effect.

If the physician is very busy and it is difficult to make an appointment, then you may be able to obtain an appointment sooner if you and the older adult are willing to accept the opinion and the examination given by the nurse practitioner.

One of the main reasons that many treatments don't work is due to the failure to communicate effectively with health care workers.Like all professional service providers, physicians tend to remember assertive patients, and outcomes are usually more successful.

A good physician/patient relationship is based on mutual respect and understanding. The physician should allow the patient to have an active role in deciding when to seek medical attention, whether to accept his advice, or to seek a second opinion. In turn, the patient owes the physician honesty and cooperation. Do not accept it if the older adult's physician attributes any of the problems to old age.

If becoming an assertive and knowledgeable consumer concerning health care and medical treatment does not sit well with your physician, then change physicians. It is vitally important that the older adult or their advocate seek the best medical treatment available. It can mean the difference between life and death.

Hospitalizations

Record all recent hospitalizations, include trips to the hospital emergency room or urgent care centers. This gives the medical professionals information that is necessary to better understand the primary health problems of the older adult. By knowing what treatment was undertaken and the results, it helps them provide the most appropriate care.

Hospitals can be scary places. Entering a hospital can mean taking risk and a loss of control. The older adult (or you) will need to fill out many forms requiring much of the personal information that you have filled out in Chapter Two of this book. Keep several copies of that information on hand for emergency hospital visits and unexpected trips to the physicians' offices.

As the primary caregiver, you will need to be the older adult's advocate and stay informed about tests, treatments, and other procedures that are being done; and to stay in close contact with the physicians and nurses. If the older adult is confused or too weak to tell medical personnel what their health problems are, then your involvement is even more essential.

You need to be cognizant that problems can occur in hospitals and that the overworked or understaffed personnel can and do make mistakes.

Hospitalization(s)

Record all within last 12 months, beginning with the most recent.

Hospital ____________________

Date Admitted __________ Length of stay __________

Reason for admission ____________________

____

Hospital ____________________

Date Admitted __________ Length of stay __________

Reason for admission ____________________

____

Hospital ____________________

Date Admitted __________ Length of stay __________

Reason for admission ____________________

____

Hospital ____________________

Date Admitted __________ Length of stay __________

Reason for admission ____________________

____

Medications

Keeping an accurate record of all medication is imperative. An estimated thirty percent of all Medicare hospital admissions are related to mistakes in medication.

Medication and its management are critical to the caregiving of an older adult. A physician who has not studied geriatrics may not know how to medicate an older and aging body. As individuals age, physical changes take place including, slower metabolism, dietary habits may contain too much sugar and/or fat, and the older adult may become more sedentary. These factors contribute to medications remaining in the aging body and bloodstream for longer periods of time, often contributing to toxicity or overmedication. To be a well-informed caregiver you need to stay up-to-date on the medications your older adult is ingesting. List all medications, including prescription drugs (Rx), over-the-counter (OTC) medications, vitamins, laxatives, and herbal remedies.

Name	Dosage	Frequency	Reason

How are the medications taken?

Specifically, can the older adult remember to take medications at the correct time, open bottle caps and lids, swallow pills, apply ointment, put in eye drops, measure liquid amounts, or inject medication?

Answer Yes or No to each of the following:

Does the Older Adult

Yes No

_____ _____ Take medications independently?

_____ _____ Take medication without assistance, but with difficulty?

Yes **No**

_____ _____ Need supervision, reminding or medication set up by another?

_____ _____ Needs hands on assistance from another?

_____ _____ Takes no medication at all?

Explain each **Yes** below

____

____

____

____

When an older adult has more than one physician, several medications can be prescribed without the physicians consulting one another, which increases the probability and risk of negative medication interactions.

Is the date on any Rx or OTC medication more than one year old?

Yes _____ No _____

If Yes, record the information from the prescription label for future reference.

Rx# or OTC	Physician	Dosage	Frequency

Now dispose of these medications permanently!

Allergic reactions/ side effects

Herbal remedies are becoming a popular trend. Many of these can be helpful, however they can be harmful if used simultaneously with certain prescription or over-the-counter medications that have been ordered for the same symptoms

To which medications, if any, is the older adult allergic?

____

____

____

____

What medications, if any, cannot be taken due to side effects such as depression, lowered blood pressure, skin rash, etc?

____

____

____

____

Sensory Abilities

All five senses decline with age. Vision usually begins to change in one's forties. Hearing impairment can begin at anytime and also with age. It is more frequent among older men than women.

The sense of smell diminishes, which means the smell of gas leaking may be a potential hazard. Many aging persons are not aware of odors on their body and may be unaware of the need to bathe or change undergarments.

The acuity of one's taste buds diminishes. Sometimes when an older adult says the food does not taste good, they mean it does not taste the same.

The decline in the sense of touch is realized by the older adult's increasing sensitivity to heat and cold. They are hotter in the summer and colder in the winter, and far more susceptible to hypothermia. Also the sweat glands cause less evaporation, making the older adult seemingly less thirsty, therefore they must be encouraged to drink water, even when they tell you they are not thirsty.

Please list any impairment in vision, hearing and/or speech (Describe the level of impairments and any aids used to improve them).

____

____

Dietary preferences

Types of foods usually consumed ______________________

____

____

____

Dislikes what kinds of foods ________________________

____

____

Dietary needs

Diabetic ___ Low sodium ___ Low cholesterol ___ Pureed ___

Low fat ___ Other __________________

Describe the older adult's appetite (from small to big eater) ________

____

Chronic Illnesses

High blood pressure ___ Managed with diet ___ Medications ___

Arthritis ___ Managed with exercise ___ Medications ___

Diabetes ___ Managed with diet ___ Oral medications ___ Insulin ___

Congestive heart failure ___ Medications ___

Other chronic illness ______________________________

____

How is this chronic illness managed? ______________________________

____

Any permanent disabilities? (Describe)

____

____

____

____

Any allergies? (Food, animals, dust, plant pollen, etc)

____

____

____

____

____

Activities of Daily Living (ADLs)

These are the performance activities that enable an older adult to maintain oneself and continue to live independently. These activities are bathing, dressing, feeding, grooming, bladder/bowel continence, toileting, transferring in and out of chair or bed and ambulating (walking). The rating scale and descriptions will help the primary caregiver, family members, and paid care providers realistically determine the tasks and care necessary to maintain the older adult in both comfort and safety. Use the following numbers and descriptive guidelines to rate the older adult's capabilities.

- ❑ 1 = Able to perform activity independently
- ❑ 2 = Able to perform activity with difficulty and more slowly
- ❑ 3 = Needs verbal reminders to perform and complete activity
- ❑ 4 = Needs hands on physical assistance to complete activity
- ❑ 5 = Unable to perform any aspect of activity independently

(Note any equipment currently in use or needed)

Bathing
Rating of this activity **1** ___ **2** ___ **3** ___ **4** ___ **5** ___

Describe the older adult's ability to complete all aspects of bathing/ showering, including the amount of time it takes or any safety risk involved

____

____

____

____

Current method of bathing Tub ____ Shower ____ Sponge bath ____

Is adaptive equipment used or needed, such as shower chair, grab bars, hand held showerhead? ______________________________

Dressing
Rating of this activity **1** ___ **2** ___ **3** ___ **4** ___ **5** ___

Describe how the older adult dresses and undresses, including opening and closing of drawers, selecting clothes, putting on and taking off upper and lower body garments, hose and shoes, buttoning and unbuttoning, zipping, or putting on and removing any medical appliances or prosthesis

____

____

____

Dressing does not occur, stays in same clothing or nightclothes both day and night.

____

Adaptive equipment used or needed

____

Feeding (Eat independently)
Rating of this activity **1** __ **2** __ **3** __ **4** __ **5** __

Describe how the older adult eats and drinks, including the ability to cut food, spread butter, or any difficulty chewing or swallowing

____

____

____

____

Adaptive equipment used or needed

____

____

____

Grooming
Rating of this activity **1** __ **2** __ **3** __ **4** __ **5** __

Describe how the older adult manages the activities of grooming, including combing hair, shaving, brushing teeth, or putting on makeup

____

____

____

Toileting
Rating of this Activity **1** __ **2** __ **3** __ **4** __ **5** __

Describe how the older adult gets to and from the toilet, on and off the commode, manages clothing, and cleans self after toileting

____

____

____

Adaptive equipment used or needed

____

____

Incontinence
Rating of this ability **1** __ **2** __ **3** __ **4** __ **5** __

Does the older adult have any incontinent devices such as a catheter or ostomy bag? Yes ____ No ____

If Yes, can the elder manage the device independently? Yes ____ No ____

Describe the level and frequency of incontinence of bladder, bowel or both (such as occasionally, frequently, continuously

____

____

____

Transferring
Rating of this Activity **1** __ **2** __ **3** __ **4** __ **5** __

Describe how the older adult gets in and out of bed, chair or wheelchair, and how they transfer (move in and out and from one to another)

____

____

____

Adaptive equipment used or needed

____

____

____

Walking/ Mobility/ Ambulation
Rating of this Activity **1** __ **2** __ **3** __ **4** __ **5** __

Describe precisely the older adult's ability to move around the house independently

____

____

____

Adaptive equipment used or needed

____

____

____

Instrumental Activities of Daily Living (IADLs)

These are the support activities that enable the older adult to live in their own home meal preparation, grocery shopping, housecleaning, laundry, transportation, money management, and the ability to use the telephone.

Check the following that best describes the older adult's ability to manage the specific activity.

	Needs hands-on assistance	Supervised	Independent	Independent with difficulty
Meal preparation				
Grocery shopping				
Housecleaning				
Laundry				
Transportation				
Money management				
Use of telephone				

Describe how the above activities are being accomplished at present and, if applicable, who is assisting the older adult

____

____

Since older adults often cannot accept their declining personal and physical limitations, their version of their Activities of Daily Living and Instrumental Activities of Daily Living may be somewhat different from your observations. This may be due to wishful thinking on their part, and a desire to return to a time in their life when they were in better health. They may not want to admit their need for assistance, or accept their growing dependence on others for care. Sometimes they resist accepting the needed help because they know it will cost money to provide that kind of care, other older adults may resent having someone else come in to take care of them. Sometimes the older adult may think that if the adult child or an "outsider" observes them, they will want to put them "in one of those places," i.e. a nursing home.

The older adult's safety and health maintenance should be your primary focus. If assistance and help is refused, point out the consequences of a fall, of becoming ill without anyone knowing about it, or of becoming so frail as to require their being moved into a nursing home situation.

A mentally competent adult has the right to refuse help. This is the kind of situation that can make the primary caregiver and other family members feel frustrated and helpless. It is not an easy time for anyone involved so the best choice here is to be patient and persistent.

Chapter Five

Assessing the older adult's mental status.

The mental ability of the older adult often varies from day to day, due to perhaps not feeling well, medication side effects, or just being lonely and isolated. The adjectives offered here will help you to describe the older adult's present actions and behaviors. The importance of this is to be able to distinguish from life-long personality traits and changes that may have taken place due to mental confusion, frustration with declining health, increasing dependence, or perhaps a new medication. You must be able to differentiate the cause of a behavior change in order to effectively find a solution.

Mental health, forgetfulness, and dementia are touchy and sensitive issues for all older adults. Memory loss is one of the most worrisome concerns for older adults and their families. Despite popular belief, memory loss is not a normal part of aging. All memory loss has a cause. It does not happen because one is a certain age. Some forgetfulness is normal at any age. This type of forgetfulness presents itself in short term bursts and usually doesn't get any worse. Slight confusion or occasional forgetfulness may also indicate the brain's overload in its informational storehouse.

It is important to realize that the human personality does not change with age, it is the one constant throughout one's lifespan.Illness, medication, and/or mental decline can exaggerate life-long personality traits, good and bad. What you may observe or think of as a personality change in the older adult is not due to aging but to some physical, mental, or emotional change.

Neither does intelligence decline with age. Creativity and judgment (wisdom) usually increases with age. Most of what we observe or attribute to loss of intelligence is a byproduct of the way the elderly are treated in our culture. Aging or being "a certain age" is demeaned and ridiculed. Even today, the terms "old timer's disease" or "senility" are used to denote the condition of an older adult who may be showing signs of forgetfulness or unusual behavior. Since senility is not a disease, this term is erroneous and obsolete.

Dementia, the contemporary term for memory loss, can happen at any age. Although Alzheimer's Disease is the most prevalent cause of dementia, later in life, there are a number of conditions with an equally large number of causes

Recognizing Depression.

The American Psychiatric Association list these criteria for a diagnosis of depression: Changes in appetite; disturbed sleep; motor retardation or agitation; fatigue and loss of energy; depressed mood or irritable mood; loss of interest or pleasure in usual activities; feelings of worthlessness, self-reproach, and excessive guilt; suicidal thinking or attempts; difficulty in thinking or concentrating.

that can produce similar symptoms. The two most frequent causes of incurable mental impairment are Alzheimer's Disease and multi-infarct dementia

Although the cause of Alzheimer's Disease is unknown, it is a degenerative disorder that is characterized by a specific set of physiological changes in the brain. Nerve fibers surrounding the brain's memory center become tangled, and information is no longer carried to or from the brain. Symptoms, such as forgetfulness and mood swings, begin slowly and become steadily worse, making early detection difficult.

At this time, there is no cure for this devastating disease, however, there are medications that can slow its progress. Education and assistance are available through the Alzheimer's Association at little or no cost.

Participation in a support group is an absolute necessity for families and caregivers of Alzheimer's victims. There you can learn methods that can aid you in handling difficult behaviors produced by this disease.

The second largest cause of dementia, the multi-infarct type, is the result of a series of small strokes or transient ischemic attacks (TIAs) which can destroy brain tissue. Its symptoms usually begin suddenly and may include weakness in an arm or leg, slurred speech, and dizziness. These symptoms do not last for more than a few days and sometimes the older adult may never fully recover. The older adult may improve for short periods of time until the next series of strokes causes further decline. In addition to confusion and difficulty with recent memory, symptoms may include bladder or bowel incontinence, poor balance and falling, inappropriate emotions such as crying or laughing at the wrong time, difficulty following instructions, and/or handling money. While no treatment can undo the damage that has been done, treatment to prevent additional strokes is important. The primary risk factor for multi-infarct dementia is high blood pressure. Some physicians refer to this type as vascular dementia.

Chronic alcoholism can also cause incurable mental impairment. Additionally, there are some 100 other symptoms that can mimic dementia: a minor head injury (from a fall), a high fever, poor nutrition, a urinary tract infection, inadequate nutrition, adverse drug reactions, and depression.

Depression, sometimes called pseudo-dementia, has early symptoms that mimic the symptoms of true memory loss. Depression can be a serious problem for older adults. Recognizing and acknowledging the symptoms of this curable dementia, is the first step in coping with depression. Since many older adults associate any mental disorder with craziness or insanity, and fear they may be "put away," getting them to admit feelings of depression may be a hard task to accomplish. Having other chronic physical problems may mask depression in older adults making an early diagnosis difficult.

Depression may become apparent in an inordinate concern for medical problems or cognitive changes. Many members of the older generation are unable to express negative emotions and tend to bury painful feelings. As a result, depression in older adults is manifested in memory problems, slowed cognitive processes, and poor decision-making.

Much of the depression that older adults suffer today is due to loneliness, isolation and loss of purpose. Depression is more common in older adults because of the many losses frequently suffered in a relatively short period of time: the loss of a spouse, a family member, friends, a pet, finances, housing, or physical abilities. All loss incurs some kind of grief, and the more serious the loss, the longer the grieving process.

An older adult's personality does not change with age. They are who they are throughout their lifetime; any changes need to be addressed long before the waning years.

Following loss, an individual can be expected to exhibit a variety of responses: shock, denial, anger, sadness, and guilt. If these responses are blocked, the person becomes "stuck," or unable to resolve the grief. This is the point where the older adult may descend into significant depression, which could require professional treatment with medication and/or counseling.

With so many causes of dementia, or similar symptoms, it is of utmost importance to obtain an accurate diagnosis. Correctly evaluating and diagnosing an older adult's mental status is not for the layman or for the primary caregiver. A professional geriatric assessment, which includes both a complete physical work up as well as mental and behavioral testing, needs to be performed by a board certified geriatrician or at a geriatric assessment center.

Through all stages of life, older adults, as well as you the primary caregiver, are entitled to live lives to the fullest within the limits of your capabilities and desires—and not to be put aside or dismissed because of age or physical infirmities. So seek out the best physical and mental health professional for the older adult, it will assist them in living their remaining years with satisfaction and dignity.

Personality assessment

Have there been gradual changes in personality within the last six months?

Yes ___ No ___

If Yes, briefly explain: ____

____

____

Which of the following best describes the older adult's current mental status?

Alert ___ Agitated ___ Complaining ___ Demanding ___

Confused___ Uncooperative ___ Changeable ___ Depressed ___

Suspicious/ Combative ___ Forgetful ___ Anxious ___

Fearful ___ Lethargic ___

In recent years, Medicare has determined that many of the so-called aging behaviors are due to depression and/or over medication.

Within certain guidelines, Medicare will pay for inpatient and/or out patient mental health services.

Ask the older adult's primary physician.

Has the older adult suffered any losses in the last six months?

Yes ___ No ___

If Yes, briefly explain: ____

____

____

Has the older adult ever complained about feeling depressed?

Yes ___ No ___

If yes, briefly explain: ____

____

____

Has the older adult had previous mental health problems?

Yes ___ No ___

If yes, briefly explain: ____

____

____

____

Has the older adult ever had a mental health evaluation?

Yes ___ No ___

If yes, briefly describe outcome: ______________________________

____

____

Has the older adult ever required any psychiatric help?

Yes ___ No ___

If Yes, briefly explain:

____

____

Hospitalized ____ In-patient ____ Out-patient ____ Takes medications ____

If hospitalized, describe cause: ______________________________

Date of hospitalization: ______________________________

Length of hospitalization: ______________________________

A very important aspect of determining degree of dementia is the older adult's ability to recognize you or other family members.

Does the older adult recognize you as the caregiver? Yes ___ No ___

ALZHEIMER'S DISEASE Understanding the Reality*

Not all confusion or dementia-like symptoms are Alzheimer's Disease.

Alzheimer's Disease is NOT:

- A natural part of aging.
- Easily diagnosed.
- Covered by government, Medicare, or most private insurance.
- Limited to those over age 65.
- Currently curable.

Alzheimer's Disease IS:

- A progressive, dementing, fatal brain disease.
- The fourth leading cause of death among adults in the United States.
- The cause of more than 100,000 deaths annually.
- A disease which knows no social or economic boundaries. It is found in all segments of the population.
- An emotional and financial nightmare for victims and their families.
- An economic time bomb for the decades ahead.

* Information courtesy of the Alzheimer's Association

Chapter Six

Understanding the three core options in caregiving.

In assessing the choices for care of the older adult, you will need to decide who is going to provide the majority of care, the primary caregiver, a volunteer family member, a paid care provider, or an alternative living arrangement. If you are the primary caregiver, you may be an only child, which throws all of the responsibility on to your shoulders, this can be seen as a blessing or a curse. The weight of being the sole decision maker may seem heavy at times, however, you can go about solving the challenges presented without interference from siblings. If you have one sibling or several, you may not have their cooperation. If this is the case, then you are the one who will be figuring out who will care for the older adult, however, it is wise to keep siblings informed whether they agree with your decisions or not.

Before you begin the search you need to understand that there are only three ways that an older adult can be cared for in the community:

1. The older adult can move in with you and your family, or another sibling or family member.
2. The older adult can stay in their home with personal assistance from a family member or paid care provider.
3. The older adult can relocate to an alternative living environment.

Each of the three choices has its pros and cons. Each choice will find both you and the older adult somewhat dissatisfied because, chances are, making this kind of a choice is not what either of you wanted. The older adult wants to be able to live on their own, independently, until they die peacefully in their sleep. And you did not want to see them become frail, disabled, and losing control of their physical or mental abilities. None of these situations will be perfect because the older adult's life has changed, and their life as they remembered it will never be the same again. At this point in time what you need to do is focus on making the best choice for the present situation, based on the physical and mental capabilities of the older adult.

Questions to think about when contemplating a caregiving change

- Is the older adult able to care for their home and surroundings?
- Could they manage with the purchased services of a homemaker, gardener, driver, etc.?
- Is the older adult able to manage their personal care? Can they, bath, dress, walk, use the bathroom, without jeopardizing their physical safety?
- Is the older adult forgetful, confused, depressed, and socially isolated?
- Do you know of a reliable home care agency in the older adult's community?
- Do you know of reliable and trustworthy paid caregivers that can come to the older adult's home?
- What kind of housing facilities exist in the older adult's community?
- If the older adult runs out of money, which of these facilities accept SSI or Medicaid/MediCal?

If your choice is to use community resources to provide the assistance the older adult needs, then you will need to locate the ones that fit within the health care needs and financial limitations of the older adult. There are so many choices in resource services and community facilities that this part of the caregiving may seem overwhelming. You will need to learn what each resource or service provides, explore its appropriateness for your older adult's needs, and then determine if the quality of the services provided will meet your standards. This can be an exhausting and trying process.

Every time you think you may have found the correct choice, a physician, a nurse, a shopkeeper, tells you from their own experience what they think is best. These individuals do not know your older adult's lifestyle, or personality. In talking to one friend about your dilemma, she may tell you to do this or don't do that. Meanwhile, another friend may give you an idea you had not thought of before. This leads you to explore yet another avenue, another resource, which only adds to your dilemma. And, all of these well-intentioned suggestions may be totally inappropriate for your older adult given their set of health care challenges.

You will need to explore all of the options and then use your head and examine your heart thoroughly before making one of these choices. You will need to remember your older adult's personality, behavior, and coping skills in the past, look at how those fit into the present, and think of both your future and theirs.

As much as you may love them, caring for an older adult is not easy. They are older and not as healthy. Even though at times their health problems may seem to improve, they will not return to their previous state of health and independence. So you will need to think it through clearly, keep an open mind, and obtain honest feedback from those that understand your unique caregiving situation. Search out people who can assist you in clarifying the issues with open and honest communication, such as friends, professionals, and support group participants.

Even though the choice may seem obvious, the decision to move forward on that choice will not be easy. You probably never thought you would have to make these choices on behalf of the older adult. You never imagined it could be so traumatic. Trying to decide on what is best for someone else is difficult enough, however when it is an older adult who is not feeling well, whose health is failing and in decline, it can feel like a monumental task. You may be thinking of what they would want, their likes and dislikes, what they are accustomed to in their daily living arrangements. How is the older adult going to react to the changes that are going to take place in the way they live? Which choice is best for their care? Who should care for them? Which caring environment is best for their health, safety, and well-being?

Making lifestyle choices is not easy. Making choices for an older adult who may be your parent, your spouse, or a close loved one will be stressful. It may seem as though you are taking over their life and making decisions for them. This may feel uncomfortable and disconcerting, especially if you grew up with the older adult helping you make the choices. The older adult was in charge and in control. The older adult made their own choices based on their frame of reference and their independence. Now the roles are reversed.

This role reversal takes place as you observe that the older adult is in a physical and/or mental decline and can no longer care for their home environment or themselves in a safe and comfortable manner. You may come to realize that you have been assuming more and more responsibility as they become more and more dependent, which may make you feel like you are the parent. It is this feeling of being the parent that often brings on ensuing frustration and conflict. Even though you may feel like you are a parent, you are not, and you never will be to any older adult.

At this point you may feel so overwhelmed that you want to give up and make it easy on yourself and accept the first solution that may come along. These feelings are normal for the circumstances. Not only should you explore all of the possibilities and the resources that fit within the personal needs and limitations of the older adult, you will have to assume the responsibility of making the choice. It may ease hard feelings, if the older adult is willing and able to discuss their preferences and be reasonable about the choices.

If you are becoming more and more confused and frustrated with the choices, then discuss them with other family members, or seek the expertise of a professional gerontologist, a social worker with geriatric experience, or attend a support group. This will help ease the burden of your responsibility and after the choice is made, you will find some comfort in knowing that you did your best.

SECTION I

Moving in with an adult child.

The losses that come with aging and illness are to be expected; yet accepting them can be difficult. Sensory impairments challenge the best of people. Failing eyesight often prevents night driving and daytime driving can become hazardous, too. The automobile, a symbol of independence, is no longer safe. The body is not as flexible and energy levels are lower. Grocery bags seem heavier; housework and the laundry are neglected; going up stairs and walking is slower. These losses and these frailties were not supposed to happen, most older adults expected to die before they became feeble and dependent. Medical technology has given them quantity with less quality in their remaining years.

You, as the adult child or primary caregiver may be making daily visits to the older adult's home, bringing prepared meals, and spending many hours assisting with the household chores and supervising their medications. As you leave, you reassure them that everything will be okay. Then on the way back to your home, you might begin worrying about the older adult's safety and well-being. If the older adult lives some distance away, the stress increases.

Your instinctive response, as you watch your older adult struggle with chronic illness and dependency, is to offer to have them come live with you. Although this sounds like a generous idea, it is not always the best option. In many cases it can be a tremendous mistake. Having an older adult move in with you is a serious commitment, and you need to think long and hard before making such an offer. Good intentions do not always guarantee good results.

When contemplating this kind of long-term closeness and proximity, there are many considerations: How well do you get along with the older adult at the present time? What was it like when you were younger and lived with the older adult? Were there personality conflicts? Was your father authoritarian? Was your mother passive and dependent, or demanding of your time? Personalities don't change. You and the older adult become more of who and what you are as you age.

A few more items for you to contemplate: Are you retired? Do you or your spouse have other significant work outside the home? Do you work from your home? Does your older adult understand that your work/career is vitally important to you? Does the older adult understand that your family must be your primary concern? The older adult must respect you, your family, and your privacy. While you may think that you can develop a closer relationship if they move in, it's more likely that former problems and irritations will become more pronounced when living together.

How does the rest of your family feel about the older adult moving in? Can your primary relationship withstand a significant reduction in quality time? Do any of your children (toddlers, teenagers, or young adults) live with you? Are any of your children willing to contribute their time and effort in assisting you with the older adult's care? If strong consideration is being given to this option, call a family meeting. Be open in discussing all of the issues, as a group and as individuals. Your first responsibility is to your spouse and to your children. If you and your immediate family do not come first, then resentment will arise on all sides.

When all of the questions and concerns have been discussed and answered to everyone's satisfaction, then it is time to look at the physical logistics of your home: Where would the older adult stay? Is your home large enough? Living together is easier in bigger spaces. Having a separate entrance, a private bath, and a sitting room are bonuses, yet not many homes have this luxury, does yours? If your family members are cramped into tight quarters, the day-to-day problems will be exacerbated, perhaps making privacy virtually impossible. Is your home equipped for an older, increasingly frail, and possibly disabled adult? If your home is on a large lot, then building an attached room or granny housing may be a solution.

Here are more ideas to think about: Are you and the older adult's lifestyles compatible? That is, are you a morning person and your parent a night person, or vise versa? What kind of dietary habits does the older adult have? Are meat and potatoes their standard fare or do they eat fish and vegetables? Does your older adult have a hearing impairment and watch a lot of television?Since the volume will be loud, expect to listen to a lot of their favorite programs. Although these things may sound insignificant, it is these kinds of things that can lead to antagonism and resentment.

The older adult has probably felt lonely and isolated in their previous surroundings. How much of your attention do they expect? Do they want to be entertained? Will the older adult want to go on outings and vacations with you and your family?

Does the older adult still cook? Will they want to assist you with the cooking or any household chores? What are the older adult's personal care capabilities?

Now make a checklist of how much help they will need with bathing, dressing, or walking. Do you feel comfortable leaving the older adult at home alone? Are you willing and able to provide this kind of care and supervision? Or if you cannot give the time the older adult requires, will you have to hire a paid care provider to assist them? Can you or your parent afford the cost of $14 to $20/hour for this kind of care? And then will your older adult accept the help of an outsider (paid caregiver)?

When an aging older adult, who is frail and nearing the end of life, moves into an adult child's home, there may be good intentions of filial warmth and sharing. Yet whether this move is by choice or default, the stage is also set for trouble unless rules and routines are agreed on in advance. By taking in your older adult, you are about to give up your privacy and not just to anyone but to someone who matters deeply to you. If this older adult is your parent, then they will know all the right buttons to push to get your attention, thereby instilling feelings of guilt, resentment, and anger. A look, a comment, or even a sigh, can trigger these feelings. These feelings may be from the long ago past, ones that you thought were gone forever. If this happens frequently, then join a support group to vent your feelings and gather helpful hints to assist you in this kind of living arrangement.

When your older adult moves in, you are gaining a loved one, but also one who is slowly losing independence. It will take time and patience to adjust to this reversal in roles. Although their wisdom and experience may be welcomed at times, the older adult will need to realize that they do not always know what is best, at least not for you, your family, or the way you have been living your life up to this point.

You will need to establish ground rules to help ease this transition. The following will aid you in shaping your guidelines and house rules.

Remember you have your limits. These limits mean that you will not be able to care for your older adult in the same way they cared for you. They are now an adult. Changing a diaper on a fully developed adult is not the same as changing one on an infant or young child. If this older adult cared for their parent in past years, they may be expecting the same kind of care. It is not the same and cannot be the same.

Times are different for you and them. You may have a career or a fulfilling job that you do not want to give up. Today's older adults are living longer with more chronic illnesses than ever before. They are losing their independence and need others to help them maintain their daily lives. This may bring up feelings of frustration and anger.

Who is the head of the house? The older adult may have been boss in their home, but you or your spouse are in charge of yours. There will be times when you will have to assert yourself. If the older adult interferes with your role as a spouse or parent, you will need to put a stop to it immediately. Older adults have been known to create a disruptive triangle in a long-term marriage. Be aware of these emotional minefields.

Outline your daily routine, make some rules, and assign tasks. You will need to make a list of your daily/weekly household routine.This will clarify your responsibilities to your self and your family. Do not allow yourself to become the maid or a cook. Give your older adult a chore (s) keeping their present limitations in mind, even if it's emptying the dishwasher or setting the table. In this way they can feel useful to you and themselves. Be very specific about the sharing of expenses, (telephone and utility bills, shopping), noise levels, smoking, and entertaining guests. When the older adult moves in with you they become part of the family not a guest.

Protect everyone's privacy. You will need to make sure that everyone has some privacy, that is a space where you and your parent or you can be alone. It is okay to make some of the rooms off-limits. If your parent wants to entertain guests, then you need to let them know when, where, and how. You will need to be very clear on all of these things and about going out to dinner, and on vacations. Do they come with the family or do they stay home with a paid care provider?

Choose your battles. When the tension rises (and it will), you will have to decide what you can live with and what you cannot. Everyone in the family will have to make compromises. If the television volume is an irritation, then buy earphones for the older adult. If the telephone is always busy when you need it, then have the older adult install their own line.

Establish a forum for complaints. Big or small problems will need to be brought out before they can fester and become overwhelming. You will need to decide ahead of time how complaints will be handled, giving all family members a chance to express themselves. Let everyone offer solutions, no matter how absurd they may sound.

Give it time. At first, you may have to endure some rough spots. Changes in life always take adjustment, especially for an older adult who has to give up their independence. This new living arrangement and the smoothing out process will take time. You will need to be patient, kind, but firm before making any decisions that may change the present arrangement.

Be patient with the older adult as this time of relinquishing independence is not any easier for them than it would be for you.

Know when to quit. If after giving this living arrangement a reasonable amount of time, (the time frame is up to you, anywhere from six months to a year), and the situation is not settling down and you are feeling stressed, you may need to reconsider. A good place to start is to listen to your body, your mind, and your heart. Is your health being affected? Are you and your spouse having more arguments and spending less time together? Are the children behaving poorly and staying in their rooms more than usual? Listen to your instincts and realize that this arrangement may not be working out. It is better to not wait until you are emotionally drained and physically exhausted. Look into alternative living arrangements, before you discuss any changes with the older adult. You will need to talk to the older adult about moving them from your home so they can prepare for it. Any change or transition will be smoother if it is done before resentment and anger builds to a boiling point.

This time in life is not easy for the older adult nor for you. Neither one of you expected this to happen: their dependency, their frailty, and needing assistance to manage the daily routine. Nonetheless, your spouse, your marriage, your children, and your job need a complete and whole person, not one who is fragmented and strained to the point of collapse. Yes, it happens all the time, caregiver burnout. Don't let it happen to you. Open your mind and heart to change and to other alternatives and choices. It is important to admit when you have made the wrong choice. In the long run, it is better for all.

SECTION II

The older adult remains at home.

Why do older adults want to stay in their homes? Their home is often too big, expensive to heat, a hardship to maintain, inadequate for their current needs, and may be in a deteriorating neighborhood. While you may suggest to the older adult the many valid and logical reasons for moving from their home, they may stubbornly refuse to move.

Before you give up in frustration, take a walk in their shoes for a moment. Their home is a part of their identity. Perhaps, this home was shared with a spouse and together they saved and made this home what it is: a refuge from the outside world. Maybe this is the home where you were raised and your children have come to visit. Home is the center of most older adult's lives. It's where most of their time is now spent. As their physical limitations increase, the world they have known contracts. Older adults focus more and more on their home and its memories and it remains a steadfast sentinel. While many other changes are taking place in their lives—physical, financial, emotional, health, and even family dynamics—their home, even though old and worn, remains the same. Is it any wonder the older adult wants to stay at home?

Older adults, as long as they are not a danger to themselves or others, are entitled to make their own decisions and to make their own choices. If they want to stay in their home, you can try to make it as safe as possible. If they need help to stay in their home, then you can assist them in locating the appropriate resources and services to help them remain there as long as possible.

Here are some questions you will need to ask yourself:

Do you feel the older adult is safe in their home? Yes _____ No _____

If No, why not? ____

____

Would the older adult be able to stay in their home, if certain safety improvements were made? Yes _____ No _____

More choices and options are open to the older adult if a decision is reached before a health care crisis occurs.

If Yes, which of the following?

Non-slip rugs instead of throw rugs _____ Access ramps _____

Wider door jams _____ Hallway handrails _____

Easier-access furniture _____ Smoke detectors _____

Raised toilet seats _____ Bathtub/toilet grab bars _____

Unbreakable dishes _____ Hire a gardener _____ Hire a handyman _____

Hire periodic housekeeping _____ Hire a bookkeeper to pay bills _____

Hire in-home help to: Pay bills ____ Cook ____ Laundry ____ Driving ____

Additional home care aids, such as safety bars, ramps, walkers, wheelchairs, aids for dressing, bathing, and household tasks, will make staying at home safer and easier. Several national companies offer catalogs of health care products to enhance the quality of life for the mildly to severely disabled. For additional information, inquire at your local senior center.

When the home is made as safe as possible, consider a personal emergency alarm, one that can be worn around the older adult's neck. It's convenient and offers peace of mind to all. The choices of systems vary, as do costs, so shop and compare.

As the primary caregiver, there are many considerations including: administering medications, hiring in-home health attendants, communication with other family members, financial resources, government entitlements, alternative living arrangements, and planning for the future are all part of an older adult remaining at home.

Often an older adult thinks that staying at home is staying independent, they do not seem or want to realize the amount of time and effort required to keep them there. Sometimes the amount of physical and emotional energy or financial resources necessitated by in-home living can be overwhelming.

The importance of becoming an informed caregiver and a good consumer cannot be overemphasized. Learn all you can about home safety issues and home health care.The physical aspects alone can burnout even the most well-intentioned and loving family caregiver. Often the wisest decision is to hire an in-home care provider, so the primary caregiver can offer the older adult the much-needed social and emotional support.

Does your older adult need more help than you can provide? Are you sacrificing personal time on behalf of caregiving responsibilities? Is the time you are spending in assisting your older adult, affecting your family or your job? Do you feel exhausted, and/or depressed? If you answer "yes" to any one of these, then it is time to hire an in-home care provider, someone who can provide the care needs of your older adult in their home.

Often the thought of hiring someone to help can be overwhelming. You might not know where to begin. The first thing is to decide which of the following two options to use: 1. to hire through a home care agency, or, 2. to hire an in-home care provider privately. Many families find the latter more affordable.

Although hiring through an agency may seem more expensive, it is often more practical because it eliminates much of the tedious paperwork involved in a private hire. It also provides the added of advantage of finding an immediate replacement should there be a personality conflict with the older adult, a no-show for work, or the worker's decision to quit without notice. If you plan to personally hire the in-home care provider rather than hire through an agency, you may be required to provide health insurance, workman's compensation, and pay employment taxes.

Whether hiring through an agency or privately, an important first step is to determine what kind of assistance the older adult needs.You will need to prepare a list of duties for the in-home care provider, that is, write a job description.

Some typical duties might include supervision with the activities the older adult is still able to do independently and companionship.

Although the older adult may perform some of these personal care activities at a slower pace it is important that the in-home care provider understand that this helps to maintain much needed self-esteem.

The older adult may require direct assistance with personal care activities such as bathing, dressing, feeding, transferring in and out of a chair or bed, walking, or grooming. Be sure to inform the in-home care provider of the older adult's physical and mental limitations, food preferences, and a timetable of their daily routine.The in-home care provider may also be able to drive the older adult to go shopping, run errands, and to the doctor. Other chores may include light housekeeping tasks, such as cooking, laundry, and watering houseplants and yard.

In these days and times it is not a good idea to advertise in the classified ads as too many people are looking for a home to live-in or an easy mark.

For a private hire, the job description should also include a work contract that can be signed by the employer (you) and the employee (the in-home care provider). A good work contract should include the following: name of employer and "household employee", wages and benefits, when and how payment will be made, hours of work, employee's Social security number, duties to be performed, unacceptable behaviors (smoking, drinking, children, overnight visitors, etc.) and termination guidelines (how much notice, reasons for termination, etc.) Be sure to date the documents and include the signatures of both employee and employer.

Finding the appropriate in-home care provider to fit the job description is the next step. Of course one of the best and easiest ways is to get a personal recommendation from a trusted relative or friend. Churches, synagogues, senior centers, local college career centers, especially those that have nursing or social work programs, are good places to locate in-home help.

Some non-profit community agencies maintain lists of individuals that are available to perform all kinds of household tasks. You can call the Alzheimer's Association, Rehabilitation Centers, or other non-profit resources for suggestions on where to look. You will be wise to shop around for the best service for the lowest price. Do not accept the first person that comes along out of desperation.

Interviewing the applicants is the next step. It is not necessary to interview everyone that applies in person. It will take too much of your valuable time. Much of the screening can be done over the telephone by describing the job in detail and stating specific expectations that are listed in the work contract as well as hours and wages. If the applicant is still interested and sounds acceptable, schedule a face-to-face interview.

When interviewing, ask questions about the applicant's work history, what they want out of the job, and previous experience with older adults. Find out if they have habits that might be disturbing to the household, such as smoking or watching television soap operas. Consider how the applicant presents themselves, both over the telephone and in person. Is physical appearance, appropriate dress (uniform), or ethnic background important to the older adult? These can be major roadblocks for acceptance by the older adult.

Tell the applicant about the older adult's condition, their physical and mental limitations and capabilities. An in-home care provider must know about the older adult's food preferences and its preparation, sleeping habits, and any incontinence. Observe the applicant's response to this information. Ask how they would handle specific situations or emergencies. Do not hide problems, as the applicant won't stay if the caring situation is not clarified.

Ask for at least three references, and always check them out. The in-home care provider needs to be capable and trustworthy, someone with whom the older adult and family members feel comfortable.

Immediately following each applicant, write down your first impressions of the individual you just interviewed. Consider the most qualified applicant and the comfort level you felt during the interview. Discuss the best applicants with a family member or friend. Based on the above findings, make a decision and then make an offer. Do not wait too long to call a good applicant because they are likely to find another job. If the applicant accepts, then set a time to sign the contract and begin work. Both employer and employee should have a copy of the job description and work contract. It is very important to sign the work contract because it provides you with legal protection.

As an employer of a "household employee," there are several legal considerations. First household employers should verify that their household insurance covers household employees in case of an accident.

It is also imperative that the household employer be fully informed of the legal responsibility of paying taxes for household employees. For more specific details that pertain to your older adult's situation, consult an accountant or elder law attorney.

The caregiving adult child should not be surprised if the older adult claims that the in-home care provider does not do things the way they like them done. Such a reaction is more the norm than the exception.That is why it is so important to find a caregiver that has a compatible personality. Many older adults have long standing, unchangeable biases or a hearing impairment that makes it difficult for them to understand a person with a strong accent.

SECTION III

Housing and Living Alternatives

This section will familiarize you with many housing alternatives that are available to older adults. Remember the old adage, "Home is where the heart is?" It applies to the familiarity and independence older adults associate with their personal physical domain, their home. Many older adults have great difficulty making the decision to leave their home, with all its memories of happy times. Nevertheless, when the physical body, as well as the physical domain, develop problems and begin to deteriorate it is time for you and the older adult to consider a different living arrangement.

Moving to a retirement home is one way to simplify an older adult's life, so they can have more time and energy to pursue activities that enhance a sense of well-being. Even under the best of circumstances, this is not an easy decision. It can be made easier, though, if you will realize that a change in living arrangement is more suitable to their current physical or health condition.

This section includes descriptions of each level of care as well as the variation in the personalities of each housing alternative. Often the primary caregiver or other family members choose a specific housing alternative based on cost and location, which is wise. However, the personality of the housing alternative should also be considered. A housing alternative gains its personality from its administrator, its staff, and, of utmost consideration, its present residents.What are the current residents like? Are they from a similar socioeconomic background? Are they high school or college graduates? Did they grow up in this town or city? Having something in common with some or at least one of the residents can make the transition and adjustment to this "new life" easier.

A major distinction that impacts most levels of care is "ambulatory" versus "non-ambulatory" licensing. Be sure to discuss the older adult's needs, limitations, and capabilities with the facility's staff, including dietary requirements, social interaction, level of continence, and personal preferences.

Insisting that an older adult move out of a house and into an alternative housing arrangement in order to ensure good physical care and safety is a loving act. You will need to reassure them, over and over again in different ways, that you are not abandoning them.You will need to tell them clearly and concisely that this housing alternative can provide the needed services which will allow you to able to spend more quality time and also provide you with more freedom for much needed self-renewal.

One of the most difficult and tedious decisions faced by the primary caregiver and other caring family members is the one of choosing an alternative living arrangement suitable for the needs of the increasingly dependent older adult. The amount of dependency will affect your choice of the level of care required and choosing the alternative living arrangement that can provide that level of care. Too often older adults and their family members wait until there is a crisis before they even begin to think about an alternative living arrangement.Then they make a hasty choice which may be regretted later. Planning ahead for all possibilities makes the decision of when and where to move much easier.

Community-based alternative living arrangements now offer more options as well as greater autonomy and dignity. They are usually more reasonably priced than nursing homes or hiring an in-home care provider. However, moving away from home at all is a situation that requires a lot of thought, discussion, and preparation. You will need to consider location, cost, level of care offered and its appropriateness to the needs of the older adult, as well as the personality of the facility and its residents.

Since there will be positive and negatives in any move, make a list of the pros and the cons, then rest on it. After visiting at least three locations, again discuss all aspects of the move. Include the older adult as well as other significant family members in the discussion. Some thoughts to ponder before discussing the possibility of relocating with the older adult:

Is the older adult willing to relocate? Yes ___ No ___

Does a new living arrangement fit within their budget? Yes ___ No ___

If Yes, have you discussed specific housing alternatives? Yes ___ No ___

Which ones?

Senior apartments ___ Retirement home ___

A continuing care or life care community ___ An assisted living facility ___

A residential care facility ___ A nursing home ___

Is a new living arrangement affordable to the older adult? Yes ___ No ___

Would a new living arrangement be affordable if you or other family members supplemented their income? Yes ___ No ___

How much could these family members contribute per month? $ ________

Consider the following suggestions when selecting an alternative living arrangement:

- ❑ Examine at least three facilities that offer the appropriate level of care
- ❑ Talk to the residents and families of these facilities
- ❑ Examine and compare costs of care
- ❑ Plan/secure financial arrangements
- ❑ Plan to discuss/educate all family members on this decision

Evaluate each facility that you visit using the following guidelines

- ❑ **Location**—Is the facility close to the primary physician, hospital, family, and friends?
- ❑ **Activities**—Does the facility have an activity program based on the residents needs and capabilities? (The number and diversity of activities depends on the abilities of the residents: exercise, bridge, day-trips, social events, music, or art therapy, etc.)
- ❑ **Buildings and grounds**—Is the facility well maintained, clean and attractive inside and out?
- ❑ **Safety and security**—Is the facility safe and secure? Depending on the type of facility, is there an emergency pull-cord in the bathroom and bedroom? How many entrances/exits does the facility have? How are these monitored (for example, security guards, alarms, or in-residence caregivers)? Have you checked with the county ombudsman or community licensing office about any complaints that the facility may have incurred?
- ❑ **Living quarters**—Is there adequate personal space, privacy, and ventilation for each resident? Can the resident bring in personal furnishings and mementos? Are the common areas roomy and comfortable for the number of residents? Are the door jams wide enough for wheelchairs?
- ❑ **Financial requirements**—Is the monthly fee subject to a cost of living increase? Is a deposit required? What does the monthly fee cover, (for example, linens, personal laundry, outside activities, medication management, assistance with bathing and dressing, incontinent supplies)?
- ❑ **Meals**—Are special meals available for conditions such as diabetes, low sodium diets or vegetarian needs? Can meals be brought to residents who are unable to eat in the dining room? Are nutritionally appropriate snacks readily available?
- ❑ **Medication**—Does the facility have a strong medication management program? Does the staff monitor residents on new medication for possible side effects?

- ❑ **Staff**—Does the staff pay attention to residents needs and desires? Do they treat each individual resident with respect? Depending on the facility and its level of care, what is the ratio of staff members to residents? Does the facility have frequent turnover of staff? Are you able to comfortably communicate with the staff of the facility? Are the administrators/manager of the facility accessible and approachable?
- ❑ **Family and friends**—Are family and friends able to visit or drop-in at any time? Can the resident be taken out for family events or community activities? Have you asked for references from other residents' families?

Descriptions of alternative living arrangements

The following living options represent different "levels of care," with important distinctions in each option. Two of the more important distinctions are:

1. Distinguishing between those living options for ambulatory and non-ambulatory and
2. Mentally or physically frail. It is of utmost importance that the facility's staff understand the older adult's needs and limitations in detail.

Senior Apartments—These are individual apartments for the independent older adult. They should be equipped with bathroom safety features, emergency pull cords, locked entry doors, and a receptionist who keeps tabs on the older adult's whereabouts. These units offer security, laundry facilities, and a limited number of parking spaces for those older adults who are still driving. They are usually located near shopping and transportation. Some apartment complexes may offer scheduled transportation and/or a daily communal meal for an additional charge. Although the cost varies, most are based on the affordability of those living on fixed income. Many are subsidized by HUD or various other city, county, or state government programs. Contact the Area Agency on Aging for locations and more information.

Retirement Home—This option resembles a large hotel, and houses 60 to 300 or more residents in various sized, individual living units. These units are for the independent older adult. Each unit has a private bathroom equipped with safety bars and emergency pull cords and a small kitchenette with a hot plate, a small refrigerator, and a microwave oven. The monthly rental fee includes 2–3 meals per day, weekly housekeeping, scheduled transportation, and a variety of planned activities. Although the cost varies, the majority of these are designed with moderate to high-level income adults in mind.

Assisted Living Facilities—This option has all of the amenities of a Retirement Home with the added services (ADLs) of medication management, bathing, dressing, and walking to the dining room. All of these services incur an additional cost. Since most older adults tend to wait until they have several chronic health problems before leaving their home, this means they usually need one or more of the assisted living services.

Large assisted living facilities are not for those older adults who are suffering from any kind of progressive dementia.

Residential Care Facility (RCF) or board and care home.—This option is a house in a residential neighborhood that is licensed to accommodate four to six older adults. These homes are ideal for individuals who require a protective environment with additional supervision for hygiene, medication, diet, and ambulation. Though ideal for those with dementia, not all RCFs accept those suffering from Alzheimer's Disease or confusion.

Most good RCFs do not mix the demented or confused resident with alert residents. Always inquire about the functional capabilities of residents and determine if the RCF is licensed for ambulatory and/or non-ambulatory residents. The cost varies with the location and amount of care required, such as incontinent care. Incontinent supplies are usually furnished for an extra cost.

Nursing or convalescent home—This option may be also referred to as a skilled nursing facility (SNF) and is for those older adults who require rehabilitation from surgery, stroke, or other disabling illnesses. SNFs also offer custodial care when the patient is bed bound and no longer able to provide any care for themselves, such as eating, turning over in bed, or have a feeding tube. Please be aware that Medicare pays only for the rehabilitative services deemed necessary by a physician. Medicare does not pay for custodial care. Medi-Cal or MediCaid, the state long-term care assistance programs, may cover the cost or share the costs for nursing home care, if the patient meets the financial requirements.

Life care or continuing care community—This option is a large planned residential community in a campus-like setting that offers most of the previous levels of care at one site: independent living, assisted living, RCF, and SNF. Some may offer specialized Alzheimer's units. Depending on the ambiance of this type of option, a sizable entry or endowment fee is required which guarantees the older adult resident admission to all levels of care as may be required over the remaining course of their life. An additional monthly fee covers meals, housekeeping, transportation and activities. With

The terms "independent" and "independence" in this section pertain to the older adult who can no longer perform IADLs or ADLs and feels that staying at home will preserve "independence."

However, by remaining at home alone, they are at risk.

The older adult may prefer to remain at home with the needed services being provided by family or paid caregivers.

The older adult may think of this as being "independent," but in reality they are dependent on outside care and assistance to remain at home.

So you will need to ask yourself, at what emotional or financial cost is this "independence."

each level of care the monthly fee goes up. In a life care community they are contracted to care for the older adult even if they run out of money. Of course, a thorough financial check is required before entry into a life care facility, so that the chances of people running out of money are reduced for the contracting facility. The advantages of this type of facility are security and all levels of care are available in one location.

Which is the most appropriate housing or living arrangement? Which ALF, RCF or SNF is better than others? Many factors are to be considered: the older adult's health, ability to manage living alone, cook, maintain personal hygiene, finances, the location and condition of the present home. Most importantly, what kind of assistance will the older adult need in the not-too-distant future.

Before considering any of the above-mentioned housing options, consider a consultation with a professional geriatric care manager and/or elder law attorney.They are extremely knowledgeable about the most appropriate resources and options, and the legal and financial resources that will be required to provide the most appropriate level of care.

Helping the older adult to realize, sooner rather than later, that they can make a new home in a safer and more suitable environment, if their physical and mental capacity diminishes, is well worth the effort. As with most changes involving an older adult's independence and control, it takes time, patience and tenacity.

Chapter Seven

Choosing the best option to meet the older adult's current caregiving needs.

There may come a time when you will have to implement a different caregiving choice. You will need to become familiar with the guidelines and tips included in this chapter, because they will assist you in making the best decision. Rethinking the present caregiving situation is normal. It may have become unmanageable for the older adult and for you, the primary caregiver. It may be that the older adult needs more care than you or a paid care provider can give. The current situation may have you lying awake nights worrying.

If possible, you will need to weigh the pros and cons of the present situation with the alternative choices available to you and the older adult. Proceeding in a methodical way will make this time less stressful for you.

Somehow, you hoped this day would not come. The day when you would have to reexamine your caregiving situation because it is not working out the way you had hoped it would. You may have promised the older adult that they could stay in their home or that you would be the one to carefor them. You may have feelings of anxiety about making this decision or guilt that you can no longer continue to care for the older adult. However, you may also realize that the older adult can no longer be cared for in the present manner. Perhaps the older adult has again fallen and was taken to the emergency room, and you know that this time something has to be done to insure the safety of the older adult, because they can no longer be left to their own devices. If the older adult's mental capacity has declined to where they are combative or are keeping you or the paid care provider up at night with their restlessness, then it is time to consider an alternative caregiving choice.

Many of the decisions you have made up to this point were obvious and therefore easily made. Other decisions you knew would take exploring and discussion before reaching a satisfactory conclusion. Considering the decision to hire full-time paid care or to move the older adult from their home is one of those times that require decisiveness. You may have been putting off even thinking of this event because of disagreements with your siblings and your own sadness and indecision. Although there is never a right time, it may be the best decision possible when it is clear that the older adult can no longer be cared for at home. You may have made a promise to keep them at home, only when you made that promise neither you nor the older adult could possibly have understood the amount of care that would be involved or how stressful it would be coping with their care.

You, your older adult, and the members of your family may each have individual styles for problem solving and decision-making. Hopefully, you and your family share the same style and this will make this process move along more smoothly. Some families can make decisions quickly, while others may be inconsistent and argumentative. A health care crisis, especially one involving an older adult, brings up the need to recognize a problem, find a flexible response, and the willingness to adapt to change. Since individual patterns of decision making may vary, you, the primary caregiver, will need to be the one to set the standards, which is not an easy task.

You will need to understand how your older adult and family members cope with crisis, change, and decision-making. Coping skills are usually set early in life, so be aware of the other family members involved and how they have dealt with other crisis situations, then plan your strategy. Certain families adapt easily to change and are flexible, while others are rigid and inflexible. For these latter families, this time of decision-making can become a crisis, because there is no established pattern. Family styles and methods of coping will continue through a crisis. If your family is close and works well together, you are among the fortunate few. If your family is one of those rigid and inflexible ones, in which every member has a different opinion and has "the right" solution, you may need professional support and advice to assist you in clarifying the issues.

Since you will need to make many decisions during this time of caregiving, the following pages will act as your guide so you can keep everyone informed. If you move through the steps suggested here, the process will be clarified, the outlook will grow brighter, the decisions more acceptable, and the outcome more successful.

You know from your own life experience that change is difficult. You've watched members of your family, as well as your friends, struggle with tough decisions. Change is difficult for everyone and it is even more difficult for older adults. Many losses and changes occur at this time in life that are irreversible and irreplaceable: changes in health, finances, home, work and/or a neighborhood. Losses can occur in physical abilities, mental capacity, friends, social contacts, housing, and pets.

When older adults have to make a major change due to failing health or declining mental capacity, they will have an even more difficult time adjusting. Not only are they losing their independence and control over their environment, they are losing the control over the life they have had up until now. They may have to have a paid care provider come to help them or they may have to move out of their memory-filled home. As shabby or elaborate as it may be, their house is their home, their castle, their last stronghold of control and the symbol of the better times in life.

As you proceed through the steps of decision-making, keep in mind that even though a change or move may be for the older adult's safety and protection, and your peace of mind, it will not be easy for them to accept.

To have a solid foundation from which to make a decision, you will need to seek good medical advice. This will help you solidify your case that the older adult needs more or a higher level of care. If you are having difficulty with the older adult or other family members, it may help to have the primary physician, an attorney, or a clergyman talk to them. Another good resource for feedback is their friends and peers.

Before you consider any major changes, evaluate the current living arrangement. Can the home be adapted with devices or aids that would ease the situation? Does the older adult simply need help driving, shopping or going to the doctor? Do they need to have help with personal care, such as taking a bath or shower? Are they resistant to the cost, or is it the feeling of dependency on another that is the problem? If cost is the problem, you may be able to introduce in-home help by giving them a week's worth of paid help as a gift. You can begin by giving four hours a day, two times per week. If you think dependency may be the reason for resistance, this will allow some adjustment time for the older adult. You will probably have to listen to a lot of complaints about the care provider or the new housing situation. Again, you will have to be patient.

If possible, it does help to include your older adult in the discussion regarding any changes that may need to take place. Reassure them that this decision is not carved in stone, it is a trial. Moving to another home or alternative living arrangement may take six weeks to six months for the older adult to adjust to the new environment. The adjustment time depends on the individual's coping skills.

For the older adult to compare the old environment with the new is normal and so is the complaining about the assisted living facility's food, the paid care provider's cooking, or the house cleaning service you may have hired. Whatever the older adult can find to complain about, they will. They are really saying "I don't like this situation because I am no longer in control." Their way may not have been as safe or efficient, but it was familiar and they felt self-sufficient. The new situation is no longer the older adult's way of doing it, so therefore, from their perspective, it is not as good.

Being prepared is the best solution for avoiding any of the conflicts in the decision-making process. Being prepared means discussing the help and assistance the older adult may need while he/she is still in good health. If you need a guide for this kind of a discussion you can use The Preparedness Checklist at the end of this chapter.

A direct and sensitive discussion about hopes, fears, and possible plans for the future makes the decision-making task a lot easier in times of crisis. In this way, the older adult can maintain a sense of control over their life and the decisions that affect it. Older adults have usually given a lot of thought to these kinds of issues, and are relieved when you or another concerned family member shows a genuine interest in their well-being. Knowing in advance what the older adult specifically desires will eliminate any doubts or qualms of conscience from you or those of other involved family members.

The first choice of most older adults is to remain at home.Whether they live alone or will require in-home help are delicate and difficult decisions at best. This kind of a decision generally comes down to a judgment call by the primary caregiver, and other concerned and involved family members. To add to all of this, the older adult may have a differing opinion from all of you. However, when the older adult is physically or mentally failing, then his/her opinion must be tempered with the wisdom and understanding of the family. You, the primary caregiver, will need to decide how far you can go in respecting the older adult's need for "independence," and when the time has come to take action in the best interest of the older adult and you.

If the safety and well-being of the older adult can be managed in the home, then it may be the best choice. To satisfy the older adult's wishes and desires, many families pool their resources of time, talent, and money, and are able to manage adequate care in the home.The decision to keep the individual at home depends most importantly on their physical abilities and mental frailty, and on your realistic opinion of their present capabilities and how these limitations may effect their being able to remain in their home and for how long.

Living alone and remaining "independent" is not always as ideal a situation as the older adult may anticipate. Frequently, the older adult finds that loneliness and a lack of reliable paid caregivers is a high price to pay for so-called "freedom" and remaining "independent." Without the network of a concerned and supportive family, or a primary caregiver, the older adult can become severely depressed, and too often, the hectic schedules of potentially supportive family members cause unexpected changes in visits, shopping trips, and doctor's appointments.

Moving toward a decision

Fear and isolation may lead the older adult from one extreme to another—from living alone to a nursing home placement. The older adult may unconsciously engineer such a placement by becoming overly passive and behaving in a helpless manner. Or the older adult may focus on physical complaints to such an extent that the primary caregiver, various family members, and/or the physician become convinced that moving to a nursing home is the best solution. In such a case, a better choice may be one of the several intermediate levels of care that exist between "independence" and complete institutionalization.

Although the primary caregiver and family members may struggle valiantly to keep the frail and declining older adult in a familiar environment, a time may come when neither family nor professional caregivers can provide the kind of care that is necessary. The decision to move your older adult from their home to a facility where the appropriate care can be provided may be difficult.The longer you wait, the more difficult the decision will be, and the more it limits your options to the various choices and levels of care.

When is the time for that decision? Each primary caregiver and each family's level of tolerance varies, however some turning points may be:

- If the financial means of paying for in-home paid care providers is almost depleted
- If the physical care is beyond the primary caregiver's or family's ability to cope
- If pain management is difficult to control
- If the older adult no longer recognizes the primary caregiver or other close family members.

- If the physical and emotional strain of the older adult's care is jeopardizing the health and well-being of the primary caregiver.
- If the physical disabilities of the older adult can no longer be managed at home.

When you first begin to consider the idea of moving the older adult to an alternative living arrangement, is the time to have a family discussion regarding the older adult's care. You will need to include siblings, other concerned family members, and, if possible, the older adult. If you do not include all of them, then the one or ones excluded will be the first to point out what is wrong and to blame you for the older adult's unhappiness or worsening physical/mental health.

Although an older adult may have been in declining health for months, or even years, siblings or close family members often choose to ignore the obvious. They need to realize that there may be a time very soon when the older adult will need help in carrying out their everyday activities. The practical issues of how the older adult will maintain themselves in their home or who will help them physically or financially either have not been discussed or the issue denied.

Frequently, the first time that the primary caregiver or family member faces the truth of their older adult's basic daily needs, is when they are notified by the hospital discharge planner following a health care crisis. The older adult or the family member may be told that the hospital will be discharging the patient within 24 hours. What this means is that the hospital has been notified that Medicare will no longer cover the expenses for the presenting health problem, so there is a rush to discharge the patient. The discharge planner may give you or other family members a list of nearby nursing homes, or home care agencies. Be warned that the discharge planner is probably not familiar with nor have they visited these referrals recently. Therefore it is up to you to find the one most suitable or a living arrangement that suits your standards for the older adult.

If this is the case and you do not want to hastily search for solutions, then request extra hospital days, pay for them out of pocket (very costly alternative), or temporarily take the older adult home with you, until you find the best nursing home or alternative living arrangement. If you move too soon, thinking that you will just "try out" the most convenient place and if it doesn't work out, then move the older adult, you will disrupt their life again making it harder for them to get better. It is during these times of health crisis that the older adult needs consistency and stability.

Sometimes what seems the most efficient way to resolve the current crisis may not be the most appropriate or effective way, even though the decision may seem sound. If the dependent older adult does not play a central part in the decision-making process, then there will be less effort put into making the plan work.

Steps to decision-making

1. Obtain a reliable health diagnosis and prognosis from the older adult's primary care physician.
2. Make a list of the pros and cons of each caregiving choice.
3. Locate and evaluate community resources that can provide the appropriate care to meet these needs.
4. Call a family meeting and invite all concerned family members.
5. Discuss the present situation, making the older adult's needs the primary focus.
6. Set realistic goals.
7. Keep family members up-to-date regarding any changes in the level of care required.
8. Make decisions on a trial basis.
9. Always be prepared to revise the plans.

Frequently, an older adult does not want to discuss personal finances or end-of-life issues. Yet, if not prepared ahead of time, the legal and financial consequences are costly and time-consuming. To assist those reluctant older adults, use the Preparedness Checklist on page 86 to aid them. Ask them to help you by saying, "Would you make this your gift to me?"

It is unrealistic to expect the complete cooperation of your entire family. However, you can accomplish a great deal if you take the decision-making process step-by-step. Mobilizing the family is more appropriate for some primary caregivers than for others.

If previous discussions have not brought favorable outcomes, a social worker or professional geriatric care manager can help the family by mediating the discussion of possibilities and alternative choices. Even under these circumstances, the core responsibility lies with the primary caregiver and family members working as a shared, functioning unit. If past issues threaten a caregiving situation or decision, a professional family therapist may help the family deal with past issues as well as the present concerns of the older adult and their future care.

No single choice or living alternative is without its problems. While the primary caregiver and the family can be an important source of love and concern, every year well over two million older adults who live with their families are abused, exploited, or neglected. You are probably saying, "It can't/won't happen in my family!" However, when tensions run high, or past hurts have not been healed, the overwhelming and often unrewarding task of caregiving can bring unwanted and undesirable behaviors. In situations where tensions run high, family care is not recommended.

A Preparedness Checklist for the Older Adult

1. Do they have a durable power of attorney for finances and/or health care?
2. In addition to Social Security, do they have adequate pension benefits or other income? Are they getting all the benefits to which they are entitled, such as SSI or Medicaid?
3. Do you know how to find out about benefits and how to apply for them?
4. Have they discussed their financial situation with you? With an attorney? In case of an emergency, does a trusted relative have access to their funds?
5. Have they discussed with you what is to be done in case of a catastrophic illness, which might result in physical or mental incapacity?
6. Have they made out a will? Do they have a power of attorney? Depending on the worth of their assets have they considered a Living Trust?
7. If they were to move far away from you and your family, what resources would be available to them if they became sick or incapacitated? Would they know what resources are appropriate and where to look for them?
8. If they were unable to live independently would they live with one of their children? Or are there more preferable living arrangements? Have they considered the necessary financial arrangements?
9. If they were not feeling well, to whom could they turn to for help with chores, shopping, transportation, etc.? Whom would they call? Where would they look for this kind of help?
10. Have they been able to talk about these matters with you, or a trusted relative or friend?

Chapter eight

Organizing information for the next layer of legal, medical and financial issues of the older adult.

The financial reserves and legal rights of the older adult are of utmost importance in your planning. You will need to understand the following essential information for their protection. If the financial matters and legal issues of the older adult are not put in order, many problems can occur down the road. You will need to locate and organize items like health insurance, bank accounts, monthly income, bills, and various other things that are in any way related to financial resources. This needs to be done in a timely and orderly manner so that the older adult can obtain the medical and personal care that may be needed at this time or in the near future.

Have you noticed recently that your older adult is having more difficulty living alone? Perhaps you have become aware that the day-to-day chores are being neglected, if this is so, then now is the time to broach the subject with the older adult of how important it is for you to know where to find their personal and financial information. If you have had to make decisions for the older adult during a previous health crisis, then you know the challenges you faced in locating the appropriate paperwork. Waiting until the older adult becomes incapacitated, either physically or mentally, then trying to locate important documents can be an extremely troublesome process.

You can avoid such circumstances by knowing where to find personal documents, such as income tax returns, power of attorney, their will and any medical directives, health and life insurance policies. In addition, you need to become familiar with the older adult's financial resources and obligations, including bank accounts, pension plans, annuities, investments, and real estate. If you organize this information in advance, then you can save yourself many hours of time and frustration.

Financial information

The financial issues related to caring for an older adult can be overwhelming, especially those related to health care, home care, and assisted living. Who pays the medical bills? Should the older adult buy long-term care insurance? What does Medicare cover? How do you calculate how much money will be needed to cover the cost of care? How long will the older adult need care? Is the adult child obligated to pay for the older adult's care? These issues can be mind-boggling.You may need to pay a professional to help you sort through all of the issues, to find the loopholes and avoid the roadblocks.

You may find that the older adult is reluctant to discuss financial issues. The subject of finances may be considered private and is often a touchy subject for most people. For many older adults their money and personal finances signify control, perhaps the only thing that they feel they have control over at this time. Some don't want to spend a dime for care, while others may not even realize how little they have and that what they have will not begin to cover the care that is needed. You will need to be patient in exploring the older adult's finances. However, it does need to be done, so you will need to start laying out the groundwork.

You may want to start by asking the older adult to make a list of the information that you would need in an emergency. Your older adult might want to keep the list with them, so ask for a copy for yourself. Some older adult's may want to give this list to a trusted third part, such as an attorney or accountant. Do not be offended by this, as many older adults do not want to share such information with their adult children or family members.

The list may include any or all of the following:

Important document	**Location**
Social security card	
Medicare card	
Health insurance policy	
Long term care policy	
Life insurance policy	
Bank account information	
Safety deposit box key	

Important document	Location
Will and/or living trust	
Living will/ medical directives	
Power of attorney	
Income tax returns	
Current bills	
Home or property deed(s) of sale	
Mortgage(s)	
Birth certificate	
Marriage certificate	
Divorce papers	
Credit card accounts	
Important contracts	
Inventory of personal property	
Burial plot/ vault receipt	
Funeral instructions	
Church/ clergy	

Once you have located these documents, the next step is to try to become familiar with your older adult's finances without being intrusive. Your assistance with the record keeping can be vital, as some older adults throw away important financial statements or bills. Trying to reconstruct important tax information or having to turn on utilities can be time consuming and tedious without efficient record keeping.

Other suggestions for helping to organize the older adult's finances is to ask them to set up a simple filing system for bills, include in this filing system canceled checks and monthly checking account statements. At the end of the year, you can offer to help the older adult make a list of all investments and sources of income. Set up a file to remind the older adult when a tax deadline is approaching. You may want to ask for their permission, so that you will receive a duplicate copy of their federal income tax return. You need to become knowledgeable about the older adult's state income tax requirements and to know if the older adult filed a state or local tax return as these must be reported on the federal return.

If your older adult is one of those who wants to be left alone and refuses your efforts of assistance, ask them to grant one simple request: ask them to take everything that comes in the mail during the month of January, except personal correspondence and checks, and put it into a large envelope. At the end of the month, the envelope can be sent to the accountant who prepares the taxes. If the older adult is comfortable with this, then ask them to begin a monthly routine of putting all of the mail into a large envelope so you can sort through it for "junk mail". If this does not work, then ask if you can review the bills on a monthly basis. Tell the older adult that without some knowledge, you could become lost if you should ever have to temporarily take over during an emergency.

If your older adult has come to the point where, due to physical or mental impairments, they are having difficulty keeping track of their finances, such as balancing the checkbook or paying bills on time, then one solution may be for you to take over these responsibilities. If this is what you decide to do, you may wish to check with utility companies, landlord or mortgager, and others to arrange for bills to come directly to you, or, alternatively, for you to be notified if bills aren't paid on time.You might consider setting up a joint checking account with the older adult.

Another solution could be to hire someone else to oversee the routine financial, legal, and medical paper work. Local social workers, professional geriatric care managers, accountants, or bookkeepers are good sources of references for this type of provider service. Be sure to interview the service provider, compare prices, and check with other clients before making your decision. Offering to give this type of service to your older adult may be a much-appreciated gift.

Financial emergencies

The potentially devastating impact of a catastrophic or long-term illness is a great concern for most older adults. Medicare, the federal health insurance program for the blind, disabled, and elderly, covers many basic medical expenses for people over age 65. Medicare has two parts. Medicare Part A is hospital insurance. Most people do not have to pay for Part A. Medicare Part B is medical insurance. Most individuals pay monthly for Part B.

Medicare Part A helps cover inpatient care in hospitals, critical access hospitals, and skilled nursing facilities. It also covers hospice care and some home health care. The older adult must meet certain conditions to qualify. Most individuals do not have to pay a monthly payment, called a premium for Part A, because either they do or a spouse paid Medicare taxes while thye were working.

Medicare B helps cover doctors' services, outpatient hospital care, and someother medical services that Part A does not cover, such as some of the services of physical and occupational therapists, and some home health care. Part B helps pay for these covered services and supplies when they are medically necessary and other medical costs. The older adult pays the Medicare Part B premium each month. Enrolling in Part B is the invidual's choice. If Part B is a choice, the premium is usually taken out of the ir monthly Social Security payment.

Supplemental health insurance (sometimes referred to as "Medigap") from a private company can be added to fill in the gaps in Medicare coverage. Policies can be purchased that cover the older adult's Medicare deductibles, longer hospital stays, co-payments for doctors' services, and a portion of prescription drugs. Medigap coverage is an important way to protect against catastrophic medical expenses should the older adult become ill. All Medigap policies issued since 1992 must match one of ten standard benefit plans, regardless of the insurance company, except in certain states. You and your older adult will want to understand what Medicare covers and the benefits provided by the ten Medigap insurance plans before making a purchase.

Long-term healthcare insurance is another means of paying for the long-term care that may be needed if the older adult needs care. With assisted living rates costing up to $5000 a month and nursing home care ranging from $100 to $500/day, consumer interest for purchasing long-term care insurance has risen. Today, policies offer more choices, better coverage, and are easier to understand than those of a few years ago. However, if the older adult decides to purchase a policy, advancing age, preexisting conditions, or poor health may make it very expensive (or impossible) to buy. Again, seek out the advice of a reliable insurance specialist to discuss the possibility of such a purchase.

Possible money resources

Catastrophic illness of health emergencies may arise that may require large amounts of money. Before considering liquidating income generating assets or selling the home, there might be another solution.

Life insurance may be used as a cash resource. If the older adult owns their own home, there are several ways to convert the equity into cash: a reverse annuity mortgage, deferred payment loan, or a sale leaseback. Financial assistance programs can also offer a means of paying for long-term care, if the older adult's resources have become depleted. There are various local, state, and federal programs to help with basic living expenses such a medical care, food, and housing. Older adults are frequently reluctant to accept governmental financial aid and social services. This generation of older adults worked hard to make their own way and are proud of their independence. To admit they now need financial aid, may be uncomfortable for them. If this is the case, you may need to remind them that they paid taxes to support these social programs, so they are entitled to use them.

Examples of assistance available to eligible older adults:

- Rent subsidies
- Utility company discounts
- Municipal programs established for low-income older adults
- Health fairs that provide free diagnostic screening
- Physicians who accept Medicare and Medicaid (MediCal) assignments
- Nonprofit and governmental health care providers who offer health services on a sliding scale
- The Veterans' Administration's Non-Service-Connected Pension with Aide and Attendance Program may offer some assistance for those honorably discharged veterans who meet criteria for disability and financial need
- Supplemental Security Income (SSI) paid by Social Security Administration to older adults living below the poverty level. Eligibility requirements vary from county to county and from state to state
- Supplemental Aid programs provided by state agencies in consultation with the Social Security Administration
- Food stamps, housekeeping services, home-delivered meals, home health care, and transportation. Availability and eligibility are variable from county to county and from state to state.

If you and the older adult have determined that assistance is needed, contact the Social Security Administration office and the Area Agency on Aging in your community. A social worker can tell you about which government programs and community services that could help. Most of these require meeting certain eligibility requirements, which can include age, state of health, as well as income level.

With encouragement and coaxing, it is still possible to prepare for the maybes and what ifs your older adult may face in the future. The older adult needs you at this time more than they ever have before, so suggest kindly that they can make this time easier on you and other family members by sharing their financial information. Explain how it would help you to be organized and ensure more beneficial care for them.

Although these efforts may seem intrusive or an invasion of privacy, becoming familiar with the older adult's financial information will make things easier for you and other family members in the event of short or long term incapacity.

The legal issues

As with financial issues, being informed about the necessary legal issues and documents that can protect the older adult is equally important. The time is now to find out which documents are in place and which are not. If your older adult should become incapacitated, then the doctor, the lawyer, the bank will turn to you for guidance and decisions. Dementia can happen overnight, not from Alzheimer's Disease but from a stroke. Without the proper legal documents, a durable power of attorney, and a health care proxy form, you may have to go through arduous legal proceedings to prove your older adult's incompetence and become the legal guardian.

Your older adult might tell you that you know what he/she wants so what does it matter. Well it does! Siblings may disagree as to the older adult's treatment, physicians may want to convince you of heroic measures, nursing homes may offer invasive treatments to protect themselves, while the older adult lives on without quality of life. You need to know very specifically the kind of treatment the older adult wants and, in order to protect their wishes, the proper legal documents need to be in place.

The older adult needs to have four documents in place: an up-to-date will, a durable power of attorney, a living will, and a health care proxy. Although you may need the professional assistance of an attorney, the minimal cost will guard you and your family against unnecessary and potentially bitter arguments and lengthy legal proceedings. These documents should be executed and signed right away.

The legal problems affecting older adults have become increasingly complicated in recent years and, as a result, family attorneys are not always qualified to advise about specific issues concerning the older population. In specialized areas, such as the preservation/transfer of assets to avoid spousal impoverishment when one spouse enters a nursing home, you may wish to consult with an attorney who practices in the relatively new specialty of law called "elder law." Elder law attorneys can help with issues regarding Medicaid (MediCal), Medicare, Social Security, and disability claims and appeals. By working with an elder law attorney, your older adult can maintain control over the important issues that govern personal property and the health issues regarding life or death decisions. The National Academy of Elder Law Attorneys (NAELA) is a professional organization that publishes an "Experience Registry" of members who specialize in various aspects of elder law. Many states also have programs for older adults who cannot afford an attorney. You can find out about these programs by contacting the older adult's county Area Agency on Aging (AAA).

Many older adults do not want to be a burden to their families or to the health care system.They want a quality life and a dignified end-of-life. The proper legal documents will protect their wishes and keep them in control at a time when they may not have any control or any voice as to what they want. The documents are described here in brief and are only meant as a general guideline.

A will describes an individual's assets, property, and belongings and explains how these are to be distributed after the individual dies. The majority of wills include a general bequest, leaving all assets to a spouse or dividing them equally among the children. Sometimes wills contain very definite instructions assigning certain items to specific individuals, and can also have instructions for establishing a trust. The will also names an executor who will pay the taxes and debts out of the estate and be sure that the assets are distributed in accord with the instructions of the will.

Legally, the will affects only that part of the estate that goes through probate. Anything in a trust, jointly owned, or given directly to a beneficiary named in a life insurance policy is not under the jurisdiction of the will. Be sure you know where the older adult keeps the will, amendments to the will and any letters of instructions that may accompany it. Keep it in a safe place, preferably in a strong box or at the attorney's office.A safe deposit box is not he best place to keep it, unless it is held in joint tenancy, because it can be sealed upon the owner's death.

There is a difference between a power of attorney your older adult may have arranged for a specific purpose and a durable power of attorney. **A power of attorney** is a legal document in which one individual gives another individual the authority to act on their behalf in specified types of transactions. This document terminates if the individual dies or becomes incapacitated or incompetent.

A durable power of attorney is a document that remains valid and enforceable despite incompetence or incapacity of the affected individual. This document terminates upon the death of that individual. Powers may include financial decisions such as purchasing and selling properties, making gifts, managing bank accounts, and insurance and medical decisions (for example, whether or not to use heroic medical treatments).

If the older adult should become incapacitated as the result of a stroke or other catastrophic illness, and does not have a durable power of attorney, then you and/or the older adult's family will have to go to court to have someone named as legal guardian to handle personal health issues and financial matters. Not only is this procedure costly, it can be extremely humiliating to the older adult. If your older adult has symptoms of dementia and you think that it is a matter of time before they will no longer be able to handle their own affairs, now is the time to have this document executed, while they can still understand the importance of these matters.

Advance medical directives

Advance medical directives are legal documents that put in writing the older adult's instructions about future medical care and treatments. These documents are designed to help guide medical professionals, family members, and friends should the older adult no longer be able to make medical decisions.These directives should be written with very particular choices and specific preferences in mind, so there are no misunderstandings at a later time. If the older adult becomes too confused or ill to communicate medical decisions, the doctors and other medical personnel usually confer directly with family members and rely on them to make decisions. Quite often family members disagree with each other or with the doctor, or they may not have known what the older adult wanted. A durable medical power of attorney, a living will, and a health care proxy form are legal documents that enable the older adult to explain in advance their wishes regarding medical care, and to name someone to make these decisions when they are unable to do so. These documents protect the older adult in two ways: 1) receiving unwanted treatment, and 2) giving them the right to refuse unwanted treatment. These documents also offer you and other family members guidance when making health care decisions and hopefully reduce any disputes or misunderstandings that may occur between family members and medical personnel.

These are the kinds of documents that most individuals put off until "later," because death is not a popular subject for discussion. However, the time to discuss the issues and have legal documents prepared is now. What you are really discussing is dignity. All individuals are going to die. The question is how do you want to die, on life support systems, totally unaware of your surroundings and unable to determine how you want to live or die? Executing these documents before the fact allows freedom and control in these situations.

Laws regulating medical directives vary by state, so, it's important to contact an attorney familiar with the requirements of the state in which the older adult resides, or you can call the county Area Agency on Aging, for help in putting the wishes in writing.

Three types of advance medical directives in most states are:

- A durable medical power of attorney is a document that allows the older adult to designate someone they trust to make medical decisions on their behalf, should they become incapacitated. Because this document eliminates the need for the older adult to know in advance all the decisions that may arise, it is important that they discuss the choices and feelings regarding medical decisions with the designated individual. An attorney should be consulted for help in drawing up a durable medical power of attorney.
- A healthcare proxy has the same effect as a durable medical power of attorney with one difference: an attorney is not usually required to complete the simple preprinted form. If the state in which the older adult resides has a healthcare proxy law, you can usually get the appropriate form from a hospital, medical facilities, a senior center, or the county Area Agency on Aging. The individual designated to make decisions should have a clear understanding of the older adult's wishes regarding medical treatment. Also the individual who acts as the healthcare proxy needs to become aware of the responsibility that is assumed with this document.
- A living will differs from the above legal documents in that, instead of naming another individual to make decisions, it specifically authorizes physicians to discontinue medical care under certain circumstances. This document can direct the physician to cease life-prolonging medical treatment when the older adult is unable to participate in the decision and is terminally ill, permanently unconscious, or severely brain damaged. A living will provides written instructions for the individual designated to make decisions on behalf of the older adult. An attorney can assist in preparing a living will.

The importance of having the above financial and legal documents prepared cannot be over emphasized. It protects the older adult's dignity and freedom of choice. Since this generation of older adults takes such pride in their achievements and independence, these documents allow them to remain in control until the end of their days. You, the primary caregiver, and other family members need to encourage your older adult to obtain these protections as soon as possible.

Chapter Nine

Preparing to handle end of life issues.

You will need this information upon the older adult's death. Pre-planning for death may sound morbid, but if the details and rituals are left unsettled, many unforeseen problems can occur involving disgruntled siblings, past hurts, and unfulfilled promises made by the older adult. Determining the preferences of the older adult is difficult once they are gone, especially since all family members may not agree. Having a prepaid internment plan and an agreement about how to divide up personal property all in place before death will ease this emotional time.

Thoughts of losing an older adult are sad and painful, even if the older adult is bedridden and desires death. The older adult may not have recognized you for quite sometime, yet this death will leave an empty space that cannot be refilled. Regardless of your relationship with this older adult, your life will be different. The death of a loved one is difficult to accept, the passage of time helps, yet there is still that empty place in your heart.

As the days and weeks pass, waves of sadness may wash over you.

Tears arrive at unexpected times—in a market or walking down a street. This is grief. Grief has many faces: sadness, sorrow, anger, regret, relief. Grief is the necessary process of a feeling person. Not all family members will experience it in the same way. No one can tell you how to grieve. You will have your own ways of grieving and others will have their own ways of working through the process. Allow it to happen at your pace.

Denying grief is a mistake. In the aftermath of loss, grief may be put off as you settle personal property and estate issues, however, grief has no time frame. Unexpressed, it may manifest itself as depression or illness. Eventually, grief will catch up with you. The feelings of loss that accompany the death of a loved one need to be expressed. Sometimes grief lasts for the rest of your life.

Since everyone experiences grief in a different way, some family members may be stoic, while others may think it is time to "get over it." If family members do not want to talk about the loss, then attend a support group especially defined for individuals like yourself. This is a safe place to meet others who have had the same loss experience. They will understand and help you through the process.

When the older adult is gone, family relationships and rituals may change. Previous roles may be altered or disappear. A brother or sister who disagreed about the older adult's care may be alienated. The sibling closest to Dad may form a new bond with Mom, which may threaten the relationship of another family member. This is a time when roles and relationships can change. This adjustment time will take its own course. Let it happen, and participate in it to the degree you desire.

End-of-life issues

❑ The funeral

❑ Disposition of body

❑ Burial

❑ Cremation

Have these arrangements been prepaid? Yes ___ No ___

Funeral home ______________________________

Address ______________________________

City ____________________ State __________ Zip__________

Phone ____________________ Fax ____________________

Types of service preferred ______________________________

Briefly describe service ______________________________

____

Person to conduct service ______________________________

Address ______________________________

City ____________________ State ________ Zip__________

Phone ____________________ Fax ____________________

Cemetery ____

Address ____

City ____________________ State ________ Zip__________

Phone ____________________ Fax ____________________

Pre-paid? Yes ___ No ___

The memorial

Persons to be notified upon death

Name ____

Address ____

City ____________________ State ________ Zip__________

Phone ____________________ Fax ____________________

Name ____

Address ____

City ____________________ State ________ Zip__________

Phone ____________________ Fax ____________________

Name ____

Address ____

City ____________________ State ________ Zip__________

Phone ____________________ Fax ____________________

Name ______________________________

Address ______________________________

City ____________________ State ________ Zip ________

Phone ________________ Fax ________________

Name ______________________________

Address ______________________________

City ____________________ State ________ Zip ________

Phone ________________ Fax ________________

Obituary text:

____

____

____

____

____

____

____

____

____

____

____

____

____

____

____

____

Which newspapers, journals, colleges need to receive obituary?

Name ____

Address ____

City ______________________ State __________ Zip __________

Phone ______________________ Fax ______________________

Name ____

Address ____

City ______________________ State __________ Zip __________

Phone ______________________ Fax ______________________

Name ____

Address ____

City ______________________ State __________ Zip __________

Phone ______________________ Fax ______________________

Name ____

Address ____

City ______________________ State __________ Zip __________

Phone ______________________ Fax ______________________

Name ____

Address ____

City ___________________________ State _________ Zip___________

Phone __________________________ Fax __________________________

Music ____

Flowers ____

Additional Notes or Comments (Favorite charities or charitable giving alternatives to flowers, etc.) ____

____

____

____

Notes ____

____

____

____

____

____

____

Chapter Ten

Supplemental reading. These articles were written by the author and published in The Quarterly Newsletter of Caregiving Solutions.

You may find these supplementary readings a help toward a better understanding of the older adult and your role as a caregiver. These articles are the outgrowth of the personal experiences of many caregivers like yourself who asked questions, sought answers, found appropriate resources, and gained acceptance of their role. When their job was finished, they were able to say they had done their best, and your best is always good enough.

Changing With Age

Personalities and Behaviors of the Elderly

Are you one of those caregiving adult children who find their parents' personality changing with the years and their frailty? Although age usually takes the blame for personality changes, it is not the culprit. A 70, 80 or 90 year old pussycat does not become a bear overnight, as an individual's basic personality is the one constant throughout life. The real culprit is the many losses that accompany aging: failing health, retirement, loss of spouse, home, friends, financial resources or favorite activities.

Life expectancy has increased appreciably during the past 30 years. For the elderly, many of these extra years lack quality and require assistance with activities of daily living (ADLs): bathing, dressing, cooking, ambulation, etc. When adult children become the caregiver and have to provide or hire care for their parents, they come face to face with many old and unresolved issues of the past. This resurrection of unfinished personal business was not an issue for previous generations, because death came quicker and earlier. Lacking experience, neither generation is prepared to cope with failing bodies and/or minds of these once strong and independent adults. Their numerous losses and changes come at a time when our aging parents are least able to cope, causing emotional behaviors that frustrate and confound the most devoted of family caregivers, as well as challenge the older parent/adult child relationship.

What are caregivers to do when faced with stubbornness and hostility, or defiance and ingratitude? These older adults cannot be punished like children, but we can lessen our frustration by learning about aging and what changes are normal. Understand that the many losses of aging can magnify a difficult personality, and interfere with the ability of well-intentioned family members to provide care. Caregivers need to distinguish between a personality style and a personality disorder. According to Wendy Lustbader, Ph.D., an individual's personality is his/her whole way of making life work—an internal state displayed in tasks, relationships, and other contexts by external behavior. Their personality allows people to feel like themselves through their actions, feelings, thoughts, and behaviors. To compensate for the many losses of aging. older adults are inclined to "turn up the volume" of their personality. People and social interactions keep them constant—their roles as spouse, parents, employees and church or community members, for example. But as roles and relationships end, the necessary affirmation of self from those outside sources diminishes and must now be self provided, causing the personality to become rigid and the traits magnified. As a result, individuals who were self centered throughout their lives become more so, and those who were generous and kind are even more likely to think of others. Erlene Rosowsky, instructor at Harvard Medical School, says that the most important part of relationships is the ability to consider other people's feelings; in other words, the ability to empathize. Many elderly are unaware of how their behaviors impact others, and are blind to their own negative behavior traits. Add in chronic illness and increasing dependency, and you get difficult personalities that are now demanding, blaming, manipulative, and exasperating.

One's personality style becomes a disorder when the individual develops traits that interfere with his/her ability to perform tasks or maintain interpersonal relationships, adds Rosowsky. Personality traits that can become disorders in older adults include:

- Chronic mistrust and suspicion (Paranoia)
- Excessive emotion and attention seeking (Histrionic Disorder)
- The need for compliments and constant validation from outside of self (Narcissism)
- Submissive, clinging behavior with a need for constant guidance and reassurance (Dependency Disorder)
- A preoccupation with details and a demand for perfection and rigid order in their environment (Obsessive Compulsive Disorder)

Personality disorders are absent of the normal give and take of social interactions and leave caregivers feeling as if they're being coerced into providing care rather than being able to give it willingly.

Unmasking and displaying of these unpleasant personality behaviors is indicated, in some, by their inability to cope with loss. For others, the changes may be related to no longer having a job in which to hide, or having lost another family member who "covered" for them. In other words, exaggerated displays of personality traits in a surviving parent may be due, not to grief, but to dad's having compensated over the years for mom's negative behaviors. Take note if a generous and outgoing individual becomes withdrawn; he/she may be suffering from depression. Fortunately, this kind of depression is treatable with counseling and medication.

Some personality disorders are the result of dementia, which is caused by organic brain changes. Often higher abstract thinking is the first to go in this kind of illness, followed by loss of inhibitions and lack of ability to self-monitor behaviors. Although loss of self control affects different personality styles in various ways, in general, aging individuals are less likely to recognize a difficult trait and hold it in check. If an individual with paranoid tendencies and short term memory loss misplaces a wallet, his/her first reaction will be to think it was stolen; the dependent individual will become fretful, tearful and ask for help; and the histrionic person will turn the house inside out to find the missing wallet. All have the same problem—only their reactions are different.

How can caregivers cope and respond to these behaviors? An excellent environment in which to discuss your parents' behavior and your reactions is within the caring and loving confidentiality of a support group. Then you will have to let go of the " golden myth," which implies that because the parent is old and nearing the end of life, he/she will become sweet, complacent, and perfect. A caregiver's realistic expectations and own stable personality can prevent the older parent from pushing buttons.

When caregiving for an older adult disintegrates into chronic criticism, hostility, or aggression, it is time to seek an outside source: a professional caregiver. This kind of stress and negative feedback is destructive and can lead to your own physical illness and/or depression. Knowing when to step aside, realizing that you cannot provide the kind of care your aging parent desires, can save not only your self esteem, but your way of life. Remember that you can only do your best at any given time, and as ffivian Greenberg says, "Your best is good enough."

Reminiscing enriches the lives of older loved ones—and ours, too.

Often in chaotic times we lose sight of our individuality and those special gifts with which we were endowed. We need to remember that each of us is individually unique. Each has a historv of personal experiences that makes us who and what we are today. We store these precious keepsakes away in our memories where we can bring them to mind throughout our lives, to contemplate in the silence of our hearts or to share with others. Reminiscing is a way of recalling these memories.

For older adults, reminiscence is often devalued and seen as a negative activity. In fact, family and friends may view it as a form of regression, a turning away from reality, a way to live in the past or even a form of mental dysfunction. Fortunately, reminiscence is now being acknowledged as having many positive effects.

Reminiscing can be a powerful resource and important coping mechanism in later years. Sharing memories can promote mental and emotional wellness, as older adults are able to preserve their identities, see their contribution to life and experience positive feelings about themselves by reviewing the joys and sorrows, successes and failures, and major and minor events of their lives. Reminiscing gives most older adults a feeling that they have indeed made a contribution to the meaning of life.

As we grow older and become more dependent on other people, including strangers, stories of what we did in the past become an important way to tell others who we are. Reminiscing is a valuable way to help older people maintain a healthy view of self. By recovering both good and bad memories, older adults can come to terms with who they are and the experiences and events that shaped their identities.

Reminiscence is a part of a larger looking back process called "life review." According to Dr. Robert Butler, chairman of the department of Gerontology, Mount Sinai Hospital and Medical School of New York, life review is a naturally occurring, universal mental process that is characterized by the progressive return to consciousness of past experiences and, particularly. the resurgence of unresolved conflicts. Reminiscence should be encouraged. As a component of the process of life review, it's curative for aging adults, parents, and relatives, and may create new levels of intimacy between generations.

In other words, reminiscing is healthy! By talking about past struggles and hardships as well as triumphs and achievements. older loved ones are able to bring meaning to the limited, often painful, lives they are currently living. Reminiscence is the process by which we make sense out of this mystery called life; it enables us to find meaning and purpose in the years we have lived.

Encourage your parents, your older loved ones, to reminisce. Push a little and have them write a journal, a chronicle or even a life review. If they cannot see or write well, have them record their stories. their histories, to pass on to succeeding generations. Where do you start? Perhaps, with pictures from the family album, or by asking how a similar experience was for them. I always find it interesting to reminisce with these wise ones: parents, older relatives, friends, and neighbors. Most of my encounters have been learning ones; I always come away with a word, a phrase, a perspective that helps me with my life challenges. Reminiscing is a way for seniors—those older adults who do not have much excitement in their current lives—to contribute to our families and us.

Most older adults benefit from reminiscence, from the active, healthy adults to those with physical, emotional and cognitive handicaps. Reminiscence especially benefits those persons suffering from Alzheimer's disease. No one is born with a perfect memory. and we all remember some things better than others. When an older adult cannot recall much about their current life, he/she may feel a sense of loneliness and disorganization. At such times, reminiscence can be used as an activity to strengthen the ability to remember.

By utilizing adult day programs, respite care and support groups, caregivers can maintain good health

According to a 1997 survey by the National Alliance on Caregiving, 22.4 million households in the United States are involved in caregiving to aging relatives and friends. An estimated 4 million of these families provide the care in their homes. The typical caregiver profile is a forty-six-year-old employed woman, who may also have a spouse and/or children. Not an easy task: eighteen to forty hours of caregiving plus a forty-hour work week! How do these caregivers manage all of their responsibilities while maintaining their own physical, mental, and spiritual health? Many of them do not—mny burn out, many become ill, some become abusers and 40% die before the care recipient. Not a pretty picture.

While there are many housing and home health care options, these long-term choices are not always appropriate or affordable for many aging adults and their families, and caregiving needs are met at home by a spouse near in age to the care recipient, or in the home of an adult child. For these at-home caregivers, adult daycare, respite care and/or a caregiver support group are invaluable resources.

Caregiving for a frail, aging relative is not easy. It's time consuming, it has a low success rate, and it is physically and emotionally exhausting. Frequently, the caregiver's duties become so all-consuming he or she fails to realize the inordinate amount of time spent on menial tasks or the repetition of questions by a loved one with dementia. This lack of self-awareness and loss of self for the sake of the care recipient's needs is hazardous to the caregivers health. The constant and ongoing act of being there for someone and having no time for oneself brings on physical illnesses such as high-blood pressure, heart attack, stroke, weight fluctuations, too much alcohol or too many pills. Depression is almost insidious to caregiving. Time-off for recreation (re-creating oneself) is necessary for the survival of a caregiver's physical and emotional well-being. Too often, the caregiver is so overwhelmed with caregiving tasks and so caught up in maintaining everyday responsibilities she or he forgets or neglects to ask for help or seek out support services that can lessen the workload. As a result, many older adults are prematurely placed in nursing homes because their caregivers have not had respite from their duties. By utilizing one or all of the resources outlined here, caregivers can lighten their duties, spend quality time with the care recipient and have more time for themselves and their families, which can only enhance the quality of life for all involved.

ADULT DAY CARE programs offer a wide range of services for adults who need a protected environment and trained staff. This type of social and physical stimulation frequently improves the older adult's behaviors while giving much needed flexibility and time-off to the caregiver to pursue his/her own work or activities. Daycare programs are often located near a multi-purpose center for active seniors, which enables them to make use of common meal and transportation services. Unlike Senior Centers, however, adult day care is usually not a "drop-in" situation, but one that requires participants to attend a regular number of days each week fora designated number of hours.

Adult Day Care is an under-utilized resource, as many families do not understand the services provided. There are two models of Adult Day Care:

1. The Social Model, which offers supervised social and educational activities including exercise, special events, nutrition, music, art, guest speakers, and family counseling; and
2. The Health Care Model, which offers similar programs to the social model with the addition of comprehensive medical treatment such as physician, nursing and rehabilitative physical, occupational and speech therapies.

When visiting a daycare program for the first time, family members often cannot believe their loved one will be better off coming here than staying home with them or a hired caregiver. What they fail to realize is that the staff is professionally trained to manage the behaviors of frail older adults whose memories or bodies are failing. In this environment, the older loved one is "normal," just like everyone else. Consequently, frustration levels will decrease, while the health and well-being of the caregiving adult child/spouse can improve dramatically as well.

With Adult Day Care, the adult child can continue working, return to a job, or participate in an activity outside the home that provides emotional and spiritual satisfaction. For the older-spouse caregiver, it offers physical and emotional relief from the twenty-four hour on-call responsibilities. According to studies at UCLA's Norman Cousins Institute, the constant and nagging stress of caregiving is often the cause of premature death to the caregiving spouse/relative in 40% of cases, because caregiving wears down the immune system. How sad, when the caregiver is so dedicated, and yet so reluctant to place the loved one in Adult Day Care.

RESPITE CARE is another support resource which offers a recess from the heavy load of caregiving. Respite can take many forms, from hiring a "sitter" one afternoon a week, to hiring someone to come in for the weekend, to taking the older adult to an assisted living, residential care or nursing facility for a weekend or even several weeks, depending on the availability of beds and their policy. Explore the opportunities of respite care, as this could truly be lifesaving in helping avoid caregiver burnout.

SUPPORT GROUPS are another valuable resource, either alone or in connection with adult day or respite care. These groups provide information about a network of aid you may be able to use, in addition to education on invaluable ways to cope. Support groups can be located at churches, community centers, hospitals, daycare centers, or nursing homes. So often caregivers wait too long to join a group, thinking they do not need one because they are managing quite well on their own, or that no one wants to hear their problems. How wrong they are! A support group allows caregivers to express their feelings in a sympathetic atmosphere. Most come to realize, usually at the first meeting, that they are not alone in the situations they face or with the kinds of reactions they feel.

Today's caregivers are pioneers. Examples of how previous generations managed the care of their older loved ones are few, because this is the longest-lived generation in human history. What's more, due to the advances in medical technology, many of today's aging adults can live up to eighteen years longer with their declining health and dementia. Caregivers need support and assistance to maintain their own good health and enjoy the many quality years ahead. Ask for help, and seek those community resources that will assist with one of the most difficult tasks you will undertake in your middle years—the care of an aging parent or loved one.

Laughter is still one of the best medicines

Many caregivers try to live up to the mythological stereotype of always having to be there for everyone. That's not realistic. Attempting to be the perfect caregiver, adult child, spouse, parent, and/or employee, can bring on feelings of disappointment and failure, which is unhealthy for all concerned. Humor and laughter is often the key to survival during these stressful times. When the idea of humor was suggested to an adult caregiving daughter, she replied, "What can I find to laugh about when I am stressed to the limit with work, kids, and my mother?" Although laughter may seem disrespectful or even sacrilegious, in the midst of caregiving, terminal illness, or approaching death, it's not.

In this hectic, frantic place of advanced technology, referred to as civilization, laughter is often forgotten. Forgotten, too, are its healing properties. Although laughter may have to be created with videos, joke books or cartoons, it can be done. All caregivers need a daily quota of laughter. It is a gift that can be freely given and received. Young children laugh and giggle hundreds of times a day. Age seems to bring on not only flabbiness of girth but of mirth, too. Humor can change that. It can make the world sane or perhaps the insanity more acceptable.

The idea of humor as medicine is not new. The *Old Testament* says, "A merry heart doeth good like medicine." Writer Norman Cousins landmark publication, *The Anatomy of An Illness,* gave impetus to humor as a healing tool. He overcame intense pain and deadly illness, using humorous books and movies. That was 30 years ago. However, it is only within the past decade that humor-as-medicine has gained respectability.

A small but growing number of hospitals have trained clowns as special visitors to patients. Intended originally for children, the infectious fun has spread throughout the hospital, to critically and terminally ill adults. Humor as an antidote for illness is being promoted throughout organizations such as the American Association of Therapeutic Humor, at conferences, workshops, on Web sites, in journals and newsletters—and a movie *Patch Adams* with Robin Williams, which is a true story. However, not all doctors have the spontaneity to kid around, as it seems a contrast to all they have learned. Perhaps they need proof that it works.

Researchers at two California universities are studying the complex biochemistry of emotions. Results suggest that "mirthful laughter" can do a lot for the human body. Not only does joking and kidding around lighten the heart and cheer the soul, it can be as therapeutic as exercise. Humor increases the heart rate, improves muscle tone, and stimulates circulation and breathing. It releases the body's endorphins, which are its natural painkillers. Some studies of humor-as-medicine have shown it lessens the need for medication and shortens recuperation time. It may even reduce stress by lowering levels of cortisol, a stress hormone that weakens the immune system, mental functions (alertness and memory) are probably stimulated as a result of rising levels of adrenaline and other chemicals that prepare the body for action. Although basic research has declined in recent years, the clinical applications have grown. People that use humor-as-medicine do not need the proof of research, they see the results daily in their work.*

Laughter can be found in caregivers support groups, where the participants have similar sounding parents. First time attendees are often surprised by the laughter and each other's stories. Upon realizing that not all of caregiving has to be serious, or the stress will win out, they join in with quips and humorous anecdotes. The sharing allows more understanding and compassion and the laughter releases tension.

On a personal note, I learned, when I worked as the social services coordinator in a hospital, to joke and kid with the patients. It lightened the seriousness of many situations. As I continued my work with older adults, I found that humor eases worries and stress, shortens generational distance and gives common ground to many family members. This lightening of feelings may encourage honesty of heart and emotional healing of past differences.

While caring for my bedridden dad last year, humor was often a release from the stress and sadness of having to watch a dignified man's physical decline and expectancy of his death. My brother and I did silly things like put on old clothes found in the chest of drawers, dancing, and miming to the music on a tape player. All of us laughed.

My dad's sense of humor would rise to the occasion and give us the impetus to do it again. His witty quips helped, too. Indicating the adult diapers, he said, "You come in wearing them and you go out wearing them." Or, when complaining of a large bruise I received from the corner of his bed, he came through with, "Try being my age (94), you bruise when you pick up your fork." The ability to laugh at oneself shows courage and strength of character. Those he had in abundance.

As Mary Poppins said, "A teaspoon of sugar makes the medicine go down, in the most delightful way." If we learn to laugh more and stress less then caregiving and the world will be a better place.

Sprituality and aging well

Spirituality is a broad term and elusive in its definition. Many associate it with religion while others think of it as an inner feeling of well-being or, as the French call it "elan," the inner spirit. The reason for attempting to attach a definition to spirituality is so research in the field of gerontology could try to understand the different ways in which individuals age, since some individuals age well while others age poorly. The thinking was that perhaps the difference is not related to one's physical health as much as it may be related to one's personal beliefs and attitude about life.

After much discussion, gerontologists arrived at the term, spiritual well-being, defined by National Interfaith Coalition on Aging as "the affirmation of life in a relationship with God, self, community, and environment that nurtures and celebrates wholeness."

David Moberg, professor emeritus of sociology at Marquette University and a major proponent of spiritual well being, has struggled with the ancient question of how God and human beings relate to each other and especially of how that relationship can be studied scientifically. He understood the complexity of measuring these dynamic issues and suggested that "spirituality flows out to all of life's relationships and concerns, merging into holistic wellness that eventuates in complete health, including security, peace, and prosperity."

Writing in *Aging Today*, Moberg's article, "Healthy Definition," says that spiritual well-being is founded in the Bible with Genesis where it states that humanity is created in the image and likeness of God. God is the great "I am," the one eternally present, who is unobservable and infinite. "Creation in God's image does not mean being identical in physical characteristics; it implies rather that each person is a spirit with a high degree of autonomy or self-direction and creativity that makes everyone unique. The 'spiritual' therefore refers to whatever is the very essence of each human being. One's spirit inevitably is implicated in everything we believe, do, and think, not in only a fraction of our behavior and thoughts. Like God, we are spirits."

For those not connected with a religious faith he puts spiritual well-being into more secular terms but the end result is the same, the very nature of humanity is spiritual. Even though "the spiritual cannot be observed directly, researchers can study its indicators, the reflections of it in people's meanings, ultimate concerns, and faith orientations, which in turn give rise to and influence their thoughts, beliefs, and actions."

Moberg compares wellness of spirit with wellness of physical growth and health. Just as the physical body needs wholesome food to grow and mature, the spirit needs wholesome spiritual nourishment. Dis-ease of the spirit can come from hypocrisy, sin, and negativity that contaminate the spirit, causing it to turn into itself, stifling growth and maturity. "Spiritual well-being therefore refers to being 'healthy' in the very core or essence of the person, regardless of one's physical and mental condition and the high or low degree of spiritual maturity already attained."

Moberg's pioneering work has influenced others in their pursuit of determining a relationship between physical health and spiritual well-being. Dr. Harold Koenig publishing in the *American Journal of Psychiatry* noted, "that religious faith by itself, independent of medical intervention and quality of life issues, can help older people recover from a serious mental disorder." In a separate study of nearly 2000 older adults in North Carolina, a research team headed by Koenig and Harvey Cohen found that those who attended religious services at least once a week were about half as likely as non-attendees to have elevated levels of interleukin-6, (an immune system protein involved in a wide array of age-related diseases). Koenig speculated that religion might influence immune functioning by enhancing coping skills, providing psychosocial support and prompting older adults to think and behave positively.

In a recent edition of *AARP Bulletin*, Herbert Benson, MD, a Harvard based cardiologist suggests "that our inner resources, particularly our spiritual beliefs, play a crucial part in an individual's well-being. He believes that human beings are "wired for God" and the very act of believing—no matter what the specific religion or philosophy--can help keep individuals well." Prayer, meditation, contemplation, and ritual are antidotes to stress and are thus good for health, according to Benson. Being a part of a congregation can be a plus, too. Worship services are full of potentially therapeutic elements—music, aesthetic surroundings, familiar rituals, prayer, and contemplation, the opportunity for socializing and fellowship."

In her book, *Making the Moments Count*, Joanne Decker states that "spiritual activities makes it possible to be in touch with one's Higher Power, express personal beliefs and values, collect thoughts, meditate, contemplate life and death, manage stress, appreciate beauty and life, and feel uplifted, motivated, and inspired." In other words, finding spiritual meaning in everyday activities can be uplifting to individuals by moving the mind away from focusing on self.

The importance of aging has been forgotten and perhaps hidden away by the focus on youth, as if old is not important or even worthless. Down through the centuries, philosophers have thought that the latter part of life is the reward for all the activity of the previous part. Yet old age is not a sedentary time or a time of idleness for the mind or the spirit. If done well, it might possibly be the biggest time for personal growth.

For many older adults who live with chronic ailments, pain, isolation, limited finances, or a terminal illness, the aging process can be difficult and dreary. Finding and expressing one's sense of spirituality can bring uplifting moments which can benefit the individual and those around them. Spirituality can be expressed through one's religion as well as other means. Joanne A. Decker's book offers many suggestions for both religion and secular spiritual activities, some others follow:

- Read spiritual materials such as The Bible, the Koran, the Talmud, and other holy books, spiritual greetings cards, classics poetry, inspirational stories, devotional books and calendars and art books.
- Pray, contemplate, and meditate.
- Listen to tapes of religious services.
- Read and write poetry
- Look at inspirational pictures: photos, posters, and art books
- Enjoy nature. Spend time in a real or imagined place.
- Listen to comforting, inspirational music.
- Keep a personal journal.
- Just be quiet.

A Caregiving Challenge: Sibling Rivalry

Families are so interesting and their dynamics can be so challenging! Families come in many varieties: natural, adoptive, step, nuclear, long-distance, estranged, close, dysfunctional, and in 57 other varieties. Each and every family is different in their histories, their customs and rituals, and yet they all contain hate, rivalry, competitiveness, indifference, alienation, and other highly charged emotions. All too often the expectations of what families are supposed to resemble are based on the images of the idealistic families created in the *Father Knows Best* or *Leave It to Beaver* sitcoms.

In reality, families are just ordinary individuals who happen to be related by blood, paper, or desire. Families are not perfect nor were they meant to be. Learning to cooperate, to cope and to find security within the bonds of family takes work. And the work of learning to get along may take months, years, or even a lifetime. This is seen all too clearly when an older parent or favorite relative faces a health crisis or becomes terminally ill. Past hurts and rivalries among family members, which may have been dormant for years and years, can be rekindled, making the care and decision making on behalf of the older adult difficult and stressful. This is called sibling rivalry, which is frequently demonstrated by the adult children of the frail older parent.

Can this be possible among mature and responsible middle-aged adult children? If there was rivalry between siblings for a parent's approval or affections when they were younger, then more than likely that rivalry still exists. This is unfinished business and although seeming immature behavior, it surfaces during times of stress and the potential loss of the parent. It can be manifested in word or action, subtle or overt, petty or gross, and is not a pretty sight. This kind of behavior can be detrimental to the appropriate care so necessary for the comfort of the older adult.

Regardless of the number of siblings in a family, usually one of them takes on the active role of primary caregiver and it's most often the daughter. Maybe she is the sibling who lives closest and has been doing most of the "caring." This daughter may visit more often, do special errands, and include mother or dad in family events. This seemingly simple routine of caring can go on for many years and may gradually increase as the parent becomes more dependent.

The remaining siblings may maintain contact with periodic visits, or by remembering birthdays and other special holidays with gifts and telephone calls. This is typical of many families. Then without warning, an older parents has a health crisis, a broken hip, a stroke, or shows signs of dementia, and the closest sibling must rally to the cause. This is often when past conflicts and unresolved issues reemerge, and competition for a parent's love and affection can interfere with appropriate choices and wise decisions.

A brother might feel as though this is his chance to be recognized as the good son and come to the aid of his mother by interfering with the recommendations of a physician or social worker. A sister, in her desire to gain the approval she never had from her mother, might offer to have mother come to live with her rather than go to "one of those places." Sibling rivalry may take the form of not making the best choices of care for a father in an attempt to save the inheritance. Another sibling may avoid expressing an opinion on a care decision or offer an impossible solution, to look like a loving child. Maybe the out-of-town brother pretends to ignore the warning telephone calls from the sibling who is the primary caregiver, and, when the parent is in the inevitable health crisis, either avoids the scene or obstructs the decisions being made. All of these behaviors are detrimental to the care so necessary at this time in the frail older parent's life. It can also place great stress on the care and decision making efforts of the primary sibling-caregiver.

Although collaborative efforts among siblings are best, they are not always possible. So what can be done to make family caregiving less stressful? Realize that not every family operates the same way. What works for one family may not work in another. Each and every family member or sibling has individual talents and liabilities. Give everyone a chance to participate. Request specific tasks of those who will fulfill them. Have realistic expectations of what is going to work in the family based on past behavior. If one sibling is going to obstruct what needs to be done, then don't involve them, but share what has to be done with the others. Whatever the family situation, communication is of utmost importance. If telephone calls are ignored or not returned, then FAX, Email, or write to that sibling about the current situation so they will stay informed. Doing this saves aggravation and stress later when the care increases or upon the death of the older parent.

Depending on the family's dynamics and the issues involved, sometimes it helps to have a third party, a geriatric care manager, social worker, elder law attorney, or clergyman mediate at a family meeting. This can help in resolving present issues. These kinds of meetings are not intended to settle issues related to past differences. At this time of stress, past issues need to be set aside as valuable time and energy is wasted on issues that may not be resolved now or ever. Siblings need to realize this and make a valiant effort to make the older parent's care their first priority.

Finding good medical care for older people

How many times have you made an appointment with your doctor for an ailment that had been bothering you for several weeks? When you finally get in to see him he greets you with, "How are you?" and your response is "Fine." I think we all have done that at one time. Many patients, especially older ones, tend to under-report specific health problems, thinking their symptoms are caused by "old age" rather than disease. While old age does affect people's health, the affect is mainly caused by them reacting differently to various diseases and drugs than younger people. These reaction changes begin around age fifty.

Regardless of age, many patients tend to assume a passive role in communicating with their physicians, perhaps because older adults, at least, are apt to view physicians as authority figures above reproach. However, if we want to receive the care and treatment best for us and our loved ones in today's medical environment of HMOs, PPOs, Managed Care and high tech tests and treatments, we absolutely must become assertive patients and take an active role in our/their health care. According to the National Institute on Aging, one of the most important parts of getting good health care is the quality of communication between you and your doctor—and, unfortunately, that is not always easy to achieve. While formerly the doctor took the lead, in today's medical system, good health care requires more of a partnership, with both patient and doctor working together to solve medical problems and maintain the patient's good health. As both a potential patient and a potential caregiver, this means asking questions if the doctor's explanations or instructions are unclear, bringing up problems even if the doctor doesn't ask, and letting the doctor know when a treatment isn't working.

The following checklist may help you or your older loved one evaluate a present doctor or locate a new one:

- Are you comfortable with the doctor? Can you openly discuss feelings and talk about personal concerns such as sexual and emotional problems?
- Does the doctor rush through every appointment with little or no conversation?
- Does the doctor listen and answer specific questions about the causes and treatments of physical problems? Or is he/she vague, impatient or unwilling to answer?
- Is time available for follow-up questions?
- Does the doctor take a thorough history and ask about past physical and emotional problems, family medical history, drugs you are taking and other matters affecting your health?
- Does the doctor attribute your problems to "old age?"
- Does the doctor have an associate to whom you can turn should he/she retire or die?

Since geriatrics, the study of medicine for older people, has only recently been introduced into medical school curriculums, not all doctors are familiar with the special needs and problems of aging. Unfortunately, too many doctors still equate aging with mental and physical decline. As a consumer, you have the right to ask questions when selecting a doctor and to expect reasonable, satisfying answers, not age-worn clichés such as "What do you expect at eighty years of age? "

A good doctor/patient relationship is based on mutual respect and communication. The doctor should allow you an active role in deciding when to seek medical attention, whether or not to accept his advice, and when to seek a second opinion. You owe the doctor your cooperation and honesty. If you feel your doctor is not giving enough answers, then find a new one. You have the righ to seek the best medical care available.

As a start toward finding a doctor who has special interest in treating older people, contact your county medical society, or state or local agency on aging. Other possible sources include referral services, medial schools, university medical centers, or the American Geriatric Society at 770 Lexington Ave #300, New York, NY 10021

Tips for communicating with the elderly

The major goal of caregiving is to gain acceptance from the care receiver with as little conflict as possible. This takes time—lots of time. The loss of independence is a major loss, and involves real change.

Be a good listener and a good communicator

- Listen attentively, even when the care receiver's words are incoherent and hard to understand. Stand or sit still and look into her or his eyes and at the lips as they talk. Move slowly and deliberately, and use a calm voice. Rushing adds to the individual's tension.
- Learn how to listen to the care receiver with interest and intelligence, particularly when it is most boring. Encourage the care receiver to talk about him or herself.
- When talking to the care receiver, speak slowly and with a pitch that is not too low or too high. Look at the person to whom you are speaking. Be patient and open-minded enough to allow the person to communicate an idea without being cut off.
- Be sensitive to frequently changing moods. Don't take hostility or irritability personally.

- Always proceed on the premise that the care receiver hears and is responsive to more than you know.
- Set a time when family and friends can phone. Calls are most appreciated. If the care receiver is hearing impaired, write short notes or letters about personal events, daily occurrences, and family concerns.
- The basic day-by-day continuity of relationships in the family provides a sense of security and satisfaction, and thus removes the underlying stress that can lower one's threshold of pain. Pleasurable stimuli including touching, stroking, comforting, loving, and smiling can sometimes compete effectively with pain.
- Always speak face-to-face with a person with impaired brain function, never from behind.
- Never ask questions that test the recollection or recognition of a care receiver with memory loss.
- Make your first words and your last words with the care receiver cheerful and pleasant.
- Be kind, understanding, gentle, and forgive. The time in the elder's life is as difficult for him or her as it is for you.

Mortality: The End of a Journey

Mortality is not easy to accept, even though death is an eventual reality for everyone. In today's feel-good, look-good culture, death is denied by not discussing it, which leaves many missing out on a very important part of life—the natural event that brings finality to having been born, walked our path, and completed a long life. Present day vernacular seems to exclude the subject of death, and attempts to eliminate the reality by using words such as passing away, demise, transition, etc. Avoidance of the word "death " is an attempt to lessen the reality, thereby making it an event to be feared rather than a natural process—one as natural as birth, aging, illness, or wellness.

In days past, particular nationalities required attending funerals and wakes, and paying respect to the inert figure of Grandpa or Auntie lying in a casket. This is difficult for a child to comprehend. The pale, still form was frightening, and an active child's imagination may have dreamt of the unrecognizable relative at rest next to the bed. For many adults, those childhood nightmares and fears are still alive. Today, we can banish our fears and know that death can be an incredible experience for the living, especially when there has been love, personal closeness, and history with a parent, spouse, or loved one.

Many frail elderly would welcome death as an escape from the indignity brought about by the loss of mental or bodily functions and/of pain. As the very old come to grips with death, they want it over with as quickly as possible. In a hurry to finish their journey, these elderly talk about dying in their sleep or taking "too many pills. " In the meantime, however, they are left with nothing to do with their time. Adult children may see it differently; they often are not ready for the finality of death. Their idea is to postpone the inevitable for as long as possible. Facing the death of a parent is a distressing reality that more times than not is avoided or denied.

In her landmark studies of death and dying, Elizabeth Kubler-Ross noted that our parents' impending death is usually accompanied by natural reactions of denial, anger, guilt, bargaining, and finally acceptance. Anger takes the form of lashing out at medical personnel, who cannot fix the parent, or even at the parent for not trying to get better. Others want to delay death with medications or heroic treatments in the futile hope the loved one will recover, when, in fact, these actions may only prolong their pain and indignity.

Acceptance and love are the keys to a comfortable experience with death. Accept that your parents' time in finite, its length known only to the Infinite, and use these precious hours, days, and weeks to prepare both yourself and your parent for their departure. Preparation for a loved one's death may sound like a morbid and uncaring act, yet if you love someone, you want their end to be as peaceful and comfortable as possible. Preparation can greatly benefit all concerned. The immediacy of putting one's house in order and completing the practical and necessary aspects needs to be emphasized. Denial at this stage is useless and detrimental.

The practical aspects of death include the complex and minute details of legal and financial matters, memorial services, burial arrangements, and disposition of personal and real property according to their wishes. Make a list, for example, of the location of valuable papers, keys, and legal documents; establish clear title on all real property; determine what treasured memento goes to which relative; plan and possibly pay for funeral arrangements prior to death, as grieving emotions affect decision-making abilities. All these issues will become your responsibility and your headache, so resolutions before the fact are imperative. Practical preparation can save a lot of unnecessary expense and trauma, as county, state, and federal regulations require minute accounting. If your parents resist, point out that they can lessen your workload and burden of responsibility by directing you to the documents and deeds necessary for settlement of their estate. Then gain their input and assistance to finalize the details.

Coming to the end of life often brings up many emotional and spiritual issues—and much unfinished business. The dying process can deeply test one's sense of self-worth and self-respect. Your parents may say they feel purposeless and burdensome. You can help them find meaning at this time by sharing a memory, a smile, a joke, a kind word. Admire them for their accomplishments, ask about the lessons they've learned and how they made it through their trials and tribulations. You will probably learn something that can bring balance to your own life. Look to find those good things for which you can honor them. Honor them for the progress they've made, because getting through life is not easy. This time of waiting for death can become a time of sharing and reviewing life's meaningful experiences and lessons learned, which is beneficial for all involved.

You can make this a time of dignity for them, an episode of peace and harmony. It is up to you. Let meaningful conversations flow naturally. For many elderly, the physical losses they have endured have made them feel helpless and fearful. Unreasonable demands for resolutions of difficult events or hurtful experiences may be futile and create anxiety, so if you have unresolved past issues, forgiving, and letting go of the hurt may be the best solution.

Your elderly parent may be eligible for Hospice, where the philosophy and practice of caring for the dying is based on the belief that death is a natural part of life. All efforts focused on enhancing whatever life remains give the family a sense of peace. Ask your physician if your parent qualifies for Hospice. If your loved on is already on Hospice and this time of dying is becoming stressfully tedious and emotional, seek out the guidance of the professionals assigned to your parent's case. These dedicated Hospice nurses and social workers are a resource of guidance and comfort to family members in their trials, tribulations, and grief. They can also assist in mediating differences among family members on caregiving issues, life-support choices, and final arrangements.

Inevitably, each individual has his or her own way of grieving. Our emotions are part of who and what we are. Support groups that focus on parental loss are available. Friends, clergy, or professional therapists can help. If you ignore or put aside your feelings, the price will be a greater sense of loss; grief is a part of loving and losing our parents. When all is said and done—the parent is laid to rest, the estate settled, and the grief is in process—focus on the good things, pleasant times, and treasured memories of the departed loved ones. Your parents gave you life and the many experiences, which are part of your journey, just as you, give to your own children. In the wise words of Sherwin B. Nuland, author of How We Die, "Death belongs to the dying and to those who love them."

Hospice: Comfort Care for the Terminally Ill and Dying

To a dying individual the past and present mean everything. Often terminal illness and impending death brings about changes in appearance, likes and dislikes. It may be difficult sometimes to realize that this individual is the same one you have known and loved throughout the years. Inside, your loved one is the same, only now they are facing three essential challenges: fear of pain, fear of loneliness, and fear of loss of control over their body and their life. Hospice can be the answer. It can assist you and the dying individual with the fears, and the challenges as well as the practical and emotional care brought about by their impending death.

Hospice is not a place but a concept that provides physical, emotional and spiritual care for the terminally ill and dying. Hospice is a very special way of caring. Hospice considers all aspects of the individual whose time is limited. The goal of hospice is to keep the individual emotionally and physically comfortable as possible by working both with the individual, the primary caregiver, family members, and paid care providers. Hospice consists of an individualized plan of care designed to help care for your loved one at home with supportive care for both the dying individual and their family.

Ideally, dying individuals should be cared for at home as they need the comfort of family, friends, and familiar possessions. However, some families feel their skills are inadequate and can become overwhelmed with the aspects of caregiving, such as: special treatments, physical care, emotional conditions, a feeling of contentment, or their fears of death and dying. These fears are normal. The Hospice program helps both the dying individual and the family understand these challenges and cope with these fears. It enhances the advantages and diminishes the problems of caring for a dying individual at home.

When medical treatment cannot cure a disease or illness, a team of hospice professionals can do a great deal by offering palliative care to reduce anxiety, control pain, and improve the quality of life. Palliative care is the aggressive treatment of physical and emotional pain and symptoms. This type of care focuses on enhancing the individual's dignity, autonomy, and quality of life, not on curing the underlying disease. The interdisciplinary Hospice team approach treats the whole person, physically, emotionally, psychologically, and spiritually. Any treatment or medication that will provide comfort for the dying individual may be considered.

The Hospice team usually consists of a doctor, nurse, social worker, home health aide, chaplain, and volunteer. Hospice personnel are carefully screened and trained to relate empathetically to the dying individual and to display genuine warmth and affection. Other specialists such as physical therapists, occupational therapists, and musical therapists may be called in as needed. The nurse will usually act as the team leader and coordinate the individual's program with the primary physician, who will monitor and supervise the plan. The team meets weekly to assess and re-evaluate the plan of care.

Hospice considers the unit of care to the dying individual and their family whomever that may be, a spouse, relatives, a life partner, and friends. One of these will be considered the primary caregiver, who then becomes an important member of the Hospice team. The primary caregiver plays a vital role in helping the team care for the dying loved one. The Hospice team provides emotional and physical support to the caregiver as well as teaching them how to give basic care. They can teach the primary caregiver about the dying process and what may be expected. The routine day-to-day care will continue to be the responsibility of the individual and the primary caregiver. It is also the responsibility of the primary caregiver and the family to notify the Hospice team leader of any changes in the individual's condition.

Anyone can refer to Hospice, however, the primary physician must certify that the dying individual has a life expectancy of six months or less. A Hospice nurse will then make a home visit to assess and evaluate the needs of the referred individual and their family. An individualized plan of care will be established to allow for changing needs or conditions, and even for the advent of new technologies. Also, an individual may leave the Hospice program at any time and for any reason.

Ninety percent of Hospice patients have a diagnosis of cancer, advanced dementia, end-stage cardiovascular disease, end-stage chronic obstructive pulmonary disease, HIV-related conditions or debility (often referred to as failure to thrive or multi-system/organ failure). Most people are uncomfortable with the idea of stopping an all-out effort to "beat " their disease. Other individuals and their families have difficulty facing death and stay in denial until death is almost imminent. Yet postponement of death with heroics or denial of the inevitable makes the end of life more difficult for all involved. Hospice should be called sooner rather than later as it offers the dying individual and their families so much in the way of physical care and emotional support.

Hospice exists to provide support and caring to individuals who are in the final phase of life and enables them to preserve their human dignity and enrich their quality of life. The role of Hospice is to support individuals in ways that are appropriate for their particular lifestyles. Hospice is available to both the rich and the poor. The costs of Hospice care are reimbursable under Medicare, Medicaid, private insurance, private payments, and other financial arrangements. Service is provided regardless of the ability to pay.

Intelligent and humane care of the dying and their loved one is one of this country's most pressing health care needs. Hospice provides a comprehensive range of services to help the dying individual and family meet the physical, emotional, and spiritual challenges faced when death is imminent. Education, training, and evaluations of Hospice services are on going activities. Attitudes toward health care in genera, and care of the dying in particular, are changing. Hospitals find terminal patients difficult to handle. A new concept was needed and Hospice fills that need.

Psychological and social challenges confronting dying individuals and their families are often more distressing than the illness and/or death. The Hospice concept affirms life, recognizing that dying is a normal process while neither hastening nor postponing death. The Hospice team assists the primary caregiver with everyday care and practical tasks. Emotional and spiritual support are available to deal with the stress and feelings of grief and loss. Hospice is designed to make the last days of life as comfortable and fulfilling as possible in an atmosphere of love and care. Hospice care offers peace of mind knowing that help is always available. It creates a compassionate environment where family members can say, "I love you " and "Goodbye."

To locate a Hospice program in your area, talk with the primary care physician, the hospital discharge planner or social worker, the state or local health department, or the state Hospice organization.

Chapter Eleven

Resources.

You will find here only some of the resources and services that are available to assist caregivers and family members with the care and responsibilities for the older adult. When family members or other volunteer help is not available or cannot meet the needs of the older adult, you may need to seek help from an agency or other service provider. Some in-home help may be covered by Medicare, Medicaid (MediCal), medical or long-term care insurance. All of the care services can be purchased. The cost of services is sometimes based on the income of the older adult. Each agency has its own fee structure, and most have minimum hours per day/per week. Be sure to clarify wages, hours, and type of insurance coverage the agency has on their employees before making final arrangements.

For the most part, service agencies and community resources are fragmented; that is, they are not all located in the same building or area of the city. In large cities, several agencies may offer the same or similar services. In rural areas, the services may be limited, or you may not find any that are appropriate. Usually, you will have to make more than one call to locate what you think is the appropriate agency, only to be confronted with a bureaucracy that gives you additional numbers to call. The search can be extremely frustrating.

Nevertheless, help is out there. You may find the right agency or the right care provider the first time but, if not, do some research. Finding the right agency to deliver the appropriate services may take a little time. You can also ask friends or neighbors for names of agencies they have used. Paid care providers often register with several agencies at once. Agencies also change management staff frequently. The Area Agency on Aging, senior centers, support groups, and local faith congregations may also have names of reputable services or agencies. Be persistent in your search.

Many Area Agencies on Aging offer a Directory of Senior Citizens Services for the area they serve, which you can obtain by calling their Community Service Agency Department. However, the directory can only be sent to those individuals over 65 years of age.

Many agencies and organizations throughout the country can also provide information and support to assist you and your older adult cope with the challenges of aging. Some are listed here. Additional resources can be found by calling your own local Area Agency on Aging or the multipurpose Senior Center nearest your older adult's home. If you are a long distance caregiver, you can call the toll-free number of the Eldercare Locator (1-800-677-1116) to find the Area Agency on Aging nearest your older adult's home town.

Federal

Social Security Administration
Office of Public inquiries
6401 Security Boulevard
Baltimore, Maryland 21235
(410) 965-1234
8 am to 5 pm, ET, Mon-Fri.
(800) 772-1213—24 hour automated service.

This federal agency operates the national retirement system and provides information on Social security coverage, earnings record, claims eligibility and adjustments, Medicare and Medicaid (MediCal in California). Under SSA is the Supplemental Security Income (SSI) program that provides additional payments to older persons already receiving public assistance. Ask for a free copy of *Your Medicare Handbook*. Individuals may file for Social security Benefits, Supplemental Security Income, State Supplemental Program (SSI/SSP), and Medicare at local offices. Each County/City has local offices to handle applications. Check local listings.

U.S. Internal Revenue Service (IRS)
(800) 829-3676
Call for addresses and other information, or check local listings.

This agency collects federal taxes. Call for a free copy of Tax Information for older Americans.

National Resources

Alzheimer's Association (ADRDA)
919 North Michigan Avenue, Suite 100
Chicago, IL 60611-1676
(800)272-3900—Toll-free helpline
8 am to 5 pm, CT, Mon-Fri

A voluntary organization that offers supportive services to patients and families coping with Alzheimer's and related disorders (Huntingtons, Picks, etc.). Use their 24-hour toll-free hotline for information on local support groups, community resources, and practical suggestions. Extensive educational materials available n patient care, research updates, diagnoses, and social services.

American Association of Retired Persons (AARP)
601 E,. Street, NW
Washington, D.C. 20049
(202) 434-2277

Helps older Americans achieve lives of independence, dignity and purpose, especially through distribution of research and information on health care, caregiving, minority issues, women's issues, and workers equity.

Children of Aging Parents (CAPS)
1609 Woodbourne Road, Suite 302A
Levittown, PA 19057-1511
(800) 227-7294

An informational resource to help adult children understand the needs and concerns of both parent and the adult child. Membership fees. CAPS has extensive national information resource files. Offered are publications on a variety of caregiving issues such as How to Find Resources in Your Area, Communication Skills, How to Plan, etc. Telephone counseling available.

Eldercare Locator Service
112-16th Street NW, Suite 100
Washington, D.C. 20036
(800) 677-1116

Nationwide assistance directory to find community assistance for seniors. Referrals are made to local organizations (usually AAA local offices) offering services to the elderly. Caliber and accuracy of information varies from area to area. Sponsored by the National Association of Area Agencies on Aging.

Health Insurance Counseling Advocacy Program (HICAP)
(800) 638-6833

Advocacy for Medicare related problems. Help with supplemental insurance purchasing, billing and claims filing. Free Service.

National Alliance for Caregiving
7201 Wisconsin Avenue, Suite 620
Bethseda, MD 20814
(310) 718-8444

A national resource center on caregiving issues, including those of the elderly. Offers information on eldercare conferences, publications, and training for family and professional caregivers.

National Association of the Area Agency on Aging
927 15th St., NW, 6th floor
Washington D.C. 20005
(202) 296-8130

This agency is responsible for planning effective use of Federal Older Americans Act fund to provide services to older Americans, generally defined as persons 60 or older. A partial list of services includes hot meals, transportation, legal aid, in-home supportive services, counseling, senior center operation, and a federally funded employment program for community service jobs for low income senior citizens. If unable to find the local number, call the number above and they will assist you.

National Association of Professional Geriatric Care Managers
1604 North Country Club Road
Tucson, AZ 85716
(520) 881-8008
8 am to 5 pm, MT, Mon-Fri.

An association of professional practitioners who arrange and oversee health-care social services for elderly and disabled clients. A call to the national office gives referrals to care managers in your area who assess the health, living conditions and needs of older adults. A geriatric care manager can also arrange and supervise all in-home help and services, and report to the family. Extremely helpful to those who are long-distance caregivers.

National Academy of Elderlaw Attorneys (NAELA)
1604 North Country Club Road
Tucson, Arizona 85716
(520) 881-4005
8 am to 5 pm, MT, Mon-Fri.

A professional association of attorneys concerned with improving the availability and delivery of legal services to older adults. NAELA maintains a national registry of attorneys who specialize in Elder Law. Write for lists by state (fee) and the free pamphlet, How to Choose an Elder Law Attorney. Also publishes brochures on legal issues affecting older adults. This office does not make referrals to individual attorneys.

U.S. Department of Veteran Affairs (Veteran Administration–VA)
Check local listings

The VA has a comprehensive system of assistance and care. Benefits for eligible veterans include nursing home care; outpatient services such as dental, prosthetic appliance and eyeglasses; alcohol and drug dependency treatment; burial and death benefits and pensions. VA hospitals offer extensive care and treatment, pharmacies and social services.

Appendix A

Health and social terms.

Area Agency on Aging (AAA)—This office is responsible for planning effective use of "Federal Older American Act" funds to provide services to older Americans, generally defined as persons 60 years or older. AAA undertakes studies regarding needs of each county's senior citizens, develops plans to meet those needs for consideration by the county's Board of Supervisors, and then administers contracts to allocate Older American Act funds to nonprofit and government entities who provide those services. A partial list of services includes hot meals, transportation, legal aid, in-home supportive services, counseling, senior center operation, and a federally funded employment program for community services job for low income seniors. AAA can also be known as the County Office on Aging.

Acute Illness—A serious illness such as a heart attack or stroke that develops rapidly with pronounced symptoms. The illness can also be of short duration such as influenza or pneumonia.

Activities of Daily Living (ADLs)—An individual's daily routine that allows him or her to maintain physical well-being, including: medications, bathing, dressing, continence, eating, grooming, toileting, and walking.

Adult Day Care Services—a daytime program of rehabilitative services and social activities for someone living at home or in an assisted living facility. Provided at a care or community center, the care usually focuses on the physically and/or mentally impaired adult, depending on the model: social daycare or health daycare. The social model offers supervised social and educational activities including exercise, special events, nutrition, music, art, guest speakers, and family counseling. The health care model offers similar recreational programs to the social model with the addition of therapeutic health services such as nursing services, rehabilitation services of physical, occupational, and speech therapies.

Assisted Living Facility (ALF)—a term used to describe large housing facilities that offer assistance services (monitoring of medications, bathing, dressing, ambulation) for older adults. The focus is on maintaining the individual's functioning and autonomy in his/her own apartment. Meals, social activities, weekly housekeeping, and scheduled transportation are included in the monthly fee.

Care Management—Assessing, arranging, and overseeing an individual's healthcare routine by a trained professional. Contact the National Association of Professional Geriatric Care Managers for a referral near you or your elderly relative.

Caregiver Support Groups—A meeting led by a professional or trained volunteer that provides a structured time for caregivers to share common concerns, express feelings, share coping skills, learn about aging issues and resources, and exchange information about caregiving. The support group leader facilitates the discussion, and provides educational and resource materials for participants. These groups can be found by calling a Senior Center, Alzheimer's Association or a local/regional hospital.

Chronic Illness—A physical or mental disability that continues or recurs frequently over a long period of time.

Continence/Incontinence—The ability or inability to voluntarily control urinary or fecal discharge.

Custodial Care—Help and supervision with activities of daily living—dressing, eating, personal hygiene and similar functions—in a residential setting.

Dementia—A clinical term used to describe a group of brain disorders that disrupt and impair cognitive functions. Cognitive functions are thinking, memory, judgment, personality, mood, and social functioning.

Discharge Planner—The professional staff member of a hospital or nursing home who develops a plan for the future care of a patient prior to discharge. This individual can provide references to agencies that offer home healthcare, board-and-care or other related options.

Do Not Resuscitate (DNR) Order—A legal document signed by the care recipient, physician, and primary (family) caregiver that expresses the elder's desire to not be given CPR or any resuscitative/reviving measures to bring back life. Since a call to 911 summons the paramedics, the care recipient will automatically be revived. If a DNR is in place, call the emergency room of the local hospital instead of 911.

Durable Power of Attorney for Health Care (DPAHC)—The DPAHC is a legally binding document that allows you to choose someone to express your health-care wishes if you are unable to do so. With a DPAHC, you maintain control over your health care. If you are incapacitated, your agent may: a) consent to treatment, b) refuse treatment, C) withdraw consent for treatment.

Geriatric Assessment Program—An evaluation of the older adult's physical, psychological, and social condition by a professional team of specialists. This team makes recommendations to the older adult, the family, and primary-care physician. Because the health problems of older individuals are frequently complex and interrelated with their social and emotional lives, this team approach to diagnosis and treatment offers a method of untangling what often proves to be interconnected health problems of seniors. A "must" for anyone suffering from symptoms of dementia.

Geriatric Care Manager (GCM)—A professional who specializes in assisting older people and their families with long-term care arrangements. A GCM has extensive knowledge about the cost, quality, and availability of services in the community. Conducts assessments or consultations to identify needs, or offers guidance in the selection of services appropriate to older adult needs.

Geriatrician—A medical doctor with special education and training in the diagnosis, treatment, and prevention of disabilities in older individuals. Geriatricians have a more holistic approach to diagnosis of older adults than many other specialists.

Geriatric Social Worker—A licensed professional who assists older adults and their families understand and cope with the social, emotional, and psychological aspects of aging. The social worker acts as coordinator, director, and teacher.

Gerontologist—An individual who, in addition to having an existing degree in nursing, social work, psychology, or social services, has received advanced training in the biological, psychological, and sociological aspects of aging.

Healthcare Proxy—A healthcare proxy has the same effect as a durable medical power of attorney with one difference: a lawyer is not usually required to complete the sample-preprinted form.

Health Insurance Counseling Advocacy Program (HICAP)—Advocacy for Medicare related problems. Helps with supplemental insurance and long-term care insurance purchasing, billing, and claims filing. Unbiased counseling. Call for comparison sheets of LTC Insurance and HMOs before purchase. Free Service. Most states have this service; however, not all are called by this title. Call your nearest AAA for specific name and phone.

Health Maintenance Organizations (HMOs)—A health plan that combines coverage of health-care costs and delivery of health care for a prepaid premium. Medicare pays the premium for those over 65 who sign up and become members with a specific HMO provider. Members receive services from personnel employed by or under contract to the HMO. HMOs generally require members/patients to select a primary-care physician (PCP) who will coordinate the patient's care. The member usually needs a referral from the PCP before he/she can go to a specialist or a hospital. Call the HICAP office near you for a comparison sheet of HMOs serving your area.

Hospice—A special way of caring for terminally ill adults and children. Hospice exists to provide support and care for individuals in the last phases of life so they might live as fully and comfortably as possible. Utilizing the expertise of Hospice in connection with the patient's physician can eliminate much of the pain/anxiety. Hospice recognizes dying as a normal process, but neither hastens nor postpones death. Medicare/HMO covers some part of the costs involved in Hospice care.

Housing Options—Alternative living arrangements including Senior Apartments, Assisted Living, Life-care, or Continuing Care Community, Intermediate Care Facility, Residential Care, Skilled Nursing Facility, AKA Nursing Home or Convalescent Home (Please see Section 7 for full descriptions).

In-Home Health Care—Qualified nurses or aides that come to the home to provide medical or personal-care services. There are several classifications: Registered or Licensed ffocational Nurse (intermittent or shift), Certified Nurses Aide, or Home Health Aide. All have had special training in various levels of care and can be hired on a shift or live-in basis. Qualifications are important, as are a compatible personality.

Instrumental Activities of Daily Living (IADLs)—Those household activities that allow an individual to maintain the basic living needs: meal preparation, shopping, transportation, and laundry.

Long-Term Care—A range of medical, nursing, custodial, social, and community services designed to help people maintain as much independence as possible within the limits of their abilities. The need for this assistance usually results from a chronic or disabling medical or physical condition.

Long-Term Care Insurance (LTC)—Insurance policies issued by private companies to assist with the costs of long-term care in nursing facilities, residential care, or in-home care. Most policies begin to pay when the beneficiary requires assistance with two ADLs. The amount and terms of coverage vary with purchase price. Call HICAP for a comparison sheet of LTC policies.

Medicare—A federal health-insurance program that helps defray many of the medical expenses of most Americans over the age of 65. Persons eligible for Social Security may also apply for Medicare benefits. Older persons should apply for Medicare benefits three months prior to their 65th birthday. For information about how to apply for Medicare, telephone, or contact the local Social Security office. Working persons over the age of 65 are entitled to Medicare even though they do not apply for Social Security. Medicare has two parts:

Part A: Hospital insurance helps pay the cost of inpatient hospital care. In some instances and under certain conditions, Part A helps pay for inpatient care in a skilled-nursing facility, for home health-care and for hospice care. Older persons and their families need to be knowledgeable about Medicare coverage. Detailed information about Medicare benefits, including a number of pamphlets explaining coverage, can be obtained from the local Social Security office.

Part B: Medical insurance helps pay for medically necessary doctor's services, outpatient hospital services and some other medical services. Enrollees must pay a monthly premium for Part B. Inquire at your local Social Security office for more information.

Medicaid (Medi-Cal in California)—A health-care program for low-income persons cooperatively financed by federal and state governments and administered by the states to eligible individuals. Benefits cover both institutional and outpatient services. However, the types of services differ from state to state. Each state has a set of criteria that establishes eligibility for services under its specific program. Further information about the Medicaid Program is available at the local county welfare, health, or social service departments or the AAA Senior Information and Referral Office.

MediGap Insurance (Supplemental Insurance Policy)—Policies sold by private insurance companies to cover the costs of services not covered by Medicare.

Ombudsman Program—Provides advocacy for older adults of long term care facilities, and information and referral to residential care facilities in areas of choice, visitation, community education, volunteer recruitment and training programs to promote quality care. Community education provides information on nursing home issues, and will counsel individuals in methods of choosing a nursing home. Advocacy coordinators accept complaints and help resolve with mediation or referral to the appropriate licensing agency.

Patient Bill of Rights—A list of policies and procedures to be followed to ensure that patients receiving healthcare services will be treated with dignity and can participate fully in decisions relevant to their healthcare.

Personal Emergency Response Systems—Equipment that monitors the safety of older adults while living at home. The older adult usually wears an activator he/she can push or squeeze when an emergency arises. The activator sends a signal to a response station, which, in turn, triggers an immediate telephone call to the older adult or a predetermined support relative, friend or neighbor. The cost of these systems varies and is usually paid for by the older adult or the family.

Physician Referral Program—A program that provides referrals to doctors specializing in geriatric medicine. The program takes into consideration not only the medical needs of older adults, but also their preferences for office location, age, gender and any foreign language requirements.

Primary Care Physician—The doctor who is consulted first when a health problem occurs and on whom the patient relies for advice, referrals and ongoing care. In HMOs' this doctor must authorize all referrals to other doctors.

Primary Caregiver—The individual who has the main responsibility for taking care of another person; usually the one who makes the decisions and organizes care and services. Each and every family has one member who is or will become the primary caregiver. This individual takes on the responsibility for making the final health, caregiving and organizational decisions on behalf of the elder. The primary caregiver does not always do the hands on caregiving.

Respite Care—Long term care services provided on a temporary basis, usually to give a much needed break to the primary caregiver(s).

Senior Citizens Information and Referral—Provides access to agencies and programs set up to help older adults. Senior Information and Referral maintains a file of information about governmental and private non profit human service programs. Services not only include information and referral but also follow up and community education to groups serving older adults. Older adults and others are encouraged to call to learn which service programs would be available to help solve a problem pertaining to a particular need.

Senior Centers —Clubs that provide social activities, information and a range of services. Many senior centers are large, publicly funded organizations that offer a wide array of activities and services including bridge, lectures, community college classes, field trips, meals, volunteer visitation, telephone reassurance, health screening, peer and legal counseling, exercise classes and both volunteer and employment opportunities. Many offer shared housing programs while others house adult daycare centers. Call the AAA to locate the nearest senior center.

Shared Housing—This program matches older citizens with other older adults or younger persons. The benefits of shared housing include reduced living costs, improved standard of living, shared household responsibilities, companionship and help in emergencies. Call AAA to find the shared housing program in your area.

Appendix B

Bibliography for caregivers.

ANOTHER COUNTRY Mary Pipher, Ph.D., The Berkley Publishing Group, New York, 2000. 325 pgs.
"Pipher explores how today's mobile, individualistic, media drenched culture prevents so many dependent old people, and the relatives trying to do right by them, from getting what they need... Her insights will help people of several generations. "

CAREGIVING FOR YOUR ELDERLY LOVED ONES, Mary Vaughn Armstrong, David C. Cook Publishing Company, Elgin, Illinois, 1990. 242 pgs.
"If you're struggling with fatigue, overload, and guilt in caring for an aging family member, here's help and encouragement."

CARING FOR THOSE WHO CAN'T, CareGiving For Your Loved One and Yourself; Carol Dettoni, Victor Books/SP Publications, Wheaton, Illinois 1993. 230 pgs.
"A Guidebook of Helpful Tips and Resources for Caregivers stressing the importance of caring for oneself. This was inspired by the author's care of her husband."

CARING FOR YOUR AGING PARENTS, A Planning and Action Guide, Donna Cohen, Ph.D. and Carl Eisdorfer, Ph.D., M.D., G.P. Putnam's Sons., New York. 272 pgs.
"One step at a time, two of America's best known experts turn caring into a manageable set of choices and provide the tools for making those choices wisely."

ELDER CARE, Family Training and Support, Amanda Smith Barusch, Sage Publications, Inc., Newberry Park, California, 1991. 196 pgs.
"Gives detailed guidelines for those interested in establishing a training program for family caregivers in addition to background material and exercises for trainers or those personally involved in caregiving."

HOSPICE CONCEPTS, A Guide to Palliative Care in Terminal Illness, Shirley Ann Smith, Research Press, Champaign, Illinois, 2000. 200 pgs.
"This book is a useful guide, and a timely reminder, of the practical principles that are the essential foundation to good hospice and palliative care."

HOW TO CARE FOR AGING PARENTS, Virginia Morris, Workman Publishing, New York, 1996. 460 pgs.
"The book that answers the questions you hoped you'd never have to ask. It's a one stop resource on the medical, emotional, legal, and financial issues involved in caring for an elderly parent."

HOW TO CARE FOR YOUR PARENTS, A Handbook For Adult Children, Nora Jean Levin, Storm King Press, Washington D.C., 1993. 110 pgs.
"This handbook offers an organized approach to gathering important information. It identifies and organizes options regarding health and long term care. Its premise is for the welfare of the whole family, the best plans are those which emerge from joint efforts."

MAKING THE MOMENTS COUNT, Leisure Activities for Caregiving Relationships, Joanne Ardolf Decker, The John Hopkins University Press, Baltimore, ML, 1997. 192 pgs.
"A valuable resource for professional caregivers, volunteers, family, and friends that provides clear strategies for making leisure part of the caregiving experience. "

REMIND ME WHO I AM, AGAIN, Linda Grant, Granta Books, London, 1998. 307 pgs.
"She offers not just a moving account of an illness (dementia), but a delicate, sensitive consideration of the relationship between memory and identity."

THE CHRISTIAN GUIDE TO PARENT CARE, Dr. Robert J. Riekse and Dr. Henry Holstege, Tyndale House Publishers, Inc., Wheaton, Illinois' 1992. 286 pgs.
"A practical resource for helping our aging parents meet their changing needs physical, emotional, spiritual."

UNDER ONE ROOF, Caring for an Aging Parent, Sheelagh McGum, Parkside Publishing, Park Ridge, Illinois, 1992. 173 pgs.
"An excellent explanation of the stress, anxiety and rewards of having your aging parent come to live in your home.

WHEN AN AGING LOVED ONE NEEDS CARE, Ron DelBene, Mary & Herb Montgomery, Upper Room Books, Nashville, TN, 1991. 32 pgs.
"A concise insight into caring with the added dimension of spirituality."

YOUR BEST IS GOOD ENOUGH: Aging Parents and Your Emotions, Vivian E. Greenberg, Lexington Books, D.C. Heath & Co., Lexington, MA, 1989. 164 pgs.
"Provides time proven strategies for coping with the conflicts and stresses inherent in caring for our elderly parents. Author offers insightful and valuable information on the needs of the elderly, the vital role emotional involvement plays in caregiving and the need for assertive and honest communication with our parents."

Educational and audiocasette programs

A BEGINNER'S GUIDE FOR CAREGIVERS OF THE ELDERLY, An Award Winning Informational Program, produced by Elana Peters, M.A., Caregiving Solutions, Irvine, CA., 1992. 2 hrs. of audio information, includes small workbook and resource booklet.
"An audio program that assists in maximizing caregiving and coping skills. A valuable tool offering practical ideas and specific steps to finding better solutions and making educated decisions."

LEGAL ISSUES AND LONG TERM CARE: Avoiding a Financial Crisis, An Award-Winning Informational Program, produced by Elana Peters, M.A.,

Caregiving Solutions, Irvine, CA, 1993. 1.5 hrs of audio information; includes small workbook and resource booklet.
"A valuable program that can assist with the legal and financial decisions associated with caregiving for an elderly relative. Offers practical ideas and guidance for protecting your elderly loved ones and preventing financial misfortune."

THE NURSING HOME DECISION: To Ease the Pain and Guilt of Placement, produced by Elana Peters, M.A., CareGiving Solutions, Irvine, CA, 1995. 40 mins.
"Ms. Peters shares her understanding, compassion and the emotional keys to help you with the most difficult decision of caregiving-placement in a long term care facility."

COMMON GROUND: Success Secrets for Caregiving and Communication with the Elderly, produced by Elana Peters, M.A, Irvine, CA, 1996, with funding from Pacific Bell Telesis. 30 mins. (Available by calling CareGiving Solutions, a non profit educational organization, (949) 253 4140.
"Ms. Peters' secrets to caregiving are invaluable to families trying to find common ground for understanding and effectively communicating with the elderly."

For aging individuals

UNDERSTANDING & IMPROVING THE INEVITABLE AGE WAVE, The Challenges and Opportunities of An Aging America, Ken Dychtwald, Ph.D., Jeremy P. Tarcher, Inc., Los Angeles, CA, 1989. 380 pgs.
"AGE WAVE will change the way Americans act today and plan for tomorrow. Every aspect of our culture is already showing signs of transformation-bringing positive new options for each of us in our work, play and social relations, and unexpected opportunities for the emergence of new products, services and businesses."

GROWING OLD, The Ultimate Freedom, Maxwell Jones, MD., Insight Books, Human Sciences Press, Inc., New York, NY., 1988. 116 pgs.
The author "encourages the freedom to contemplate, to listen, to read, and to learn what is afforded those in the later years of life. He demonstrates how these years can provide an ideal opportunity for new growth

processes, built on a lifetime of experiences and a growing awareness of new levels of reality."

HOW TO STAY ALIVE AS LONG AS YOU LIVE, Practical Guides for Christian Living, Robert H. Spain, Dimensions for Living, Nashville, TN, 1992. 142 pgs.
"Life, real life, can begin whenever you want it to begin, and it can go on and on-regardless of age. It is not living but staying alive as long as you live that is important."

REMINISCING TOGETHER, Howard I. Thorsheim, Ph.D. and Bruce Roberts, Ph.D., CompCare Publishers, Minneapolis, Minnesota, 1990. 143 pgs.
Ways to Help Us Keep Mentally Fit As We Grow Older—especially for those who are choosing to grow older with courage and imagination.

WHEN MEN GRIEVE, Why Men Grieve Differently & How You Can Help, Elizabeth Levang, Ph.D., Fairview Press, Minneapolis, Minnesota, 1998. 165 pgs.
"A helpful and insightful book about how men face loss. This book will help women to understand men in grief and help men to understand themselves."

WIDOW'S WALK, Ann Hosansky, Donald I. Fine, Inc., New York, 1993. 213 pgs.
"A story of one woman's walk through the first year and a half of widowhood, in hopes that sharing these true experiences may help others on their own journey toward survival."